T012701?

FIND YOUR SMILE

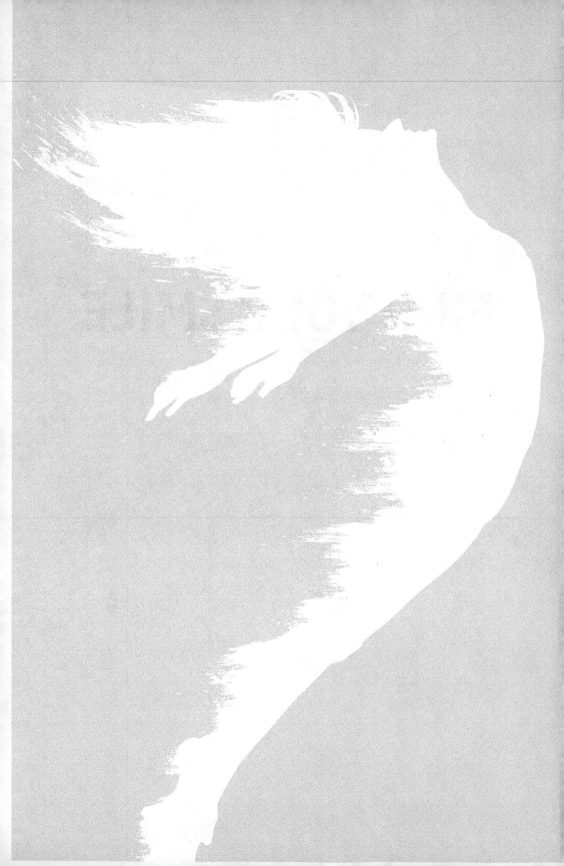

AND OUTER

HOW YOUR INNER SMILE CAN CHANGE YOUR LIFE

FIND YOUR SMILE

DR. KRISTINE WEST

Advantage.

Copyright © 2021 by Dr. Kristine West.

All rights reserved. No part of this book may be used or reproduced in any manner whatsoever without prior written consent of the author, except as provided by the United States of America copyright law.

Published by Advantage, Charleston, South Carolina.
Member of Advantage Media Group.

ADVANTAGE is a registered trademark, and the Advantage colophon is a trademark of Advantage Media Group, Inc.

Printed in the United States of America.

10 9 8 7 6 5 4 3 2 1

ISBN: 978-1-64225-181-4
LCCN: 2021902858

Cover and layout design by David Taylor.

This publication is designed to provide accurate and authoritative information in regard to the subject matter covered. It is sold with the understanding that the publisher is not engaged in rendering legal, accounting, or other professional services. If legal advice or other expert assistance is required, the services of a competent professional person should be sought.

Advantage Media Group is proud to be a part of the Tree Neutral® program. Tree Neutral offsets the number of trees consumed in the production and printing of this book by taking proactive steps such as planting trees in direct proportion to the number of trees used to print books. To learn more about Tree Neutral, please visit **www.treeneutral.com**.

Advantage Media Group is a publisher of business, self-improvement, and professional development books and online learning. We help entrepreneurs, business leaders, and professionals share their Stories, Passion, and Knowledge to help others Learn & Grow. Do you have a manuscript or book idea that you would like us to consider for publishing? Please visit **advantagefamily.com** or call **1.866.775.1696**.

To all those who are inspired to rediscover their inner smiles, and to all the women who so freely share their smiles with others while forgetting to nurture their own.

CONTENTS

FOREWORD

Kyle Mercer
Author, *Life at Altitude*

As a mentor, teacher, and coach, it is so satisfying to be able to write this foreword to Kris's book. During our relationship over nine and a half years, I've seen her commitment to her growth, freedom, and truth continue to merge and flourish.

When she first came to me, her life looked perfect. Everybody would have seen her as somebody who was successful—successful in business, with family, and in her relationships. She had set her life up seemingly perfectly, yet it wasn't satisfying. That is when she realized the difference between doing life right and doing life with heart.

Making a break and transitioning from living the life that society and culture says is the "right" one into a life of integrity, freedom, purpose, love, and heart takes great courage, and Kris has that courage. As a client and student of mine, she continually is willing to step into the zone of her own discomfort—this is the only way we can grow. We have to constantly be willing to challenge our beliefs about the world, our beliefs about ourselves, and what is true for us. It isn't always easy. Sometimes we have to face change. Kris has been determined and is determined to have a life that feels true to her.

I love that she is taking this step in her journey to write this book to share and express what she's experienced. Not only is this great for you, but this is great for her, because she gets to see how far she's come and the steps she's made in solidifying her understanding of herself, her choices, and where she is going in life.

There's something about putting it down and packaging it and handing it off that allows us to step into a new place.

I feel so honored to work with Kris, and I truly feel a deep friend-ship and kinship with her. She is one of my best students and cou-rageously takes the next step forward—she steps in, listens, receives, and reflects, and I am absolutely certain that she's never going to stop growing and learning and creating. I am really looking forward to the next step in her journey and the beauty and the freedom that she is going to create for herself.

All of my love, appreciation, and care,

Kyle

INTRODUCTION

SMILE LIKE YOU MEAN IT

If you smile when you are alone, then you really mean it.
—*ANDY ROONEY*

This year I celebrate twenty-five years of being an orthodontist, and I still love creating beautiful smiles. When I went into orthodontics, I didn't think about the amazing opportunity that I would have to provide a lasting impact on so many people's lives. My greatest joy comes from realizing that I have touched my patients' lives in ways that made them a bit happier, brought them joy, and helped them smile inside and out. Creating beautiful smiles and straightening teeth is, of course, a significant part of being an orthodontist, and I am going to provide our patients the best bites and smiles I possibly can, but more important for me is genuinely connecting with my patients, getting to know them, getting to know their stories, and meeting them where they are in their journey.

A lot of the teenagers we treat are quiet and shy when they first come in, and my team and I find ways to connect with them to make sure they know they have our full attention when they are here. Each time they come in, they are a little less shy, and the next thing we know, we often can't get them to stop talking and smiling long enough for us to look in their mouths!

Our adult patients are also occasionally hesitant or even a little skeptical when they first arrive. One of my adult patients is a professional vlogger. She spends a lot of time in front of the camera and was really embarrassed to smile and show her teeth. Her transformation was amazing. A new outer smile brightened her inner smile, and she elevated her online persona to a new level. Now her smile lights up any room she enters. It is such a joy for me to treat adult patients and have them at the end of their journeys say, "Oh my gosh, I can't believe I didn't do this sooner" or "What a difference it's made in my life."

Many orthodontists prefer not to treat adults. Adults can be difficult; it's harder to move adult teeth, and they have other dental challenges that children don't have. My practice is unusual in that many of my patients are adults, and most of those are women. I did not choose to become the orthodontist for adults; in fact, I didn't set out to be a dentist or an orthodontist at all. My journey into dentistry and then orthodontics has been an evolution.

My exposure to dentistry came at an early age. My uncle went to dental school, and I looked up to him as a hero when I was a child. Even at the young age of seven, I can still remember his dental school graduation and thinking to myself, "Wow, Uncle Jim is going to be a dentist. There must be something special about it." That thought stayed in the back of my mind.

When I was eight years old, my mother remarried. My new stepfather was our dentist, which provided me an even closer introduction to dentistry. My stepsiblings and I would spend a lot of time at his dental office; it was a fun place to be. We'd make the dental chair go up and down and pretend we were dentists. We'd check out all the prizes for the kids and grab one or two for ourselves. At sixteen, I was told I was going to be spending the rest of my high school summers working for him as an assistant.

As a teenager, of course, I didn't want to be there, and I made my feelings clear. One day my stepfather finally said, "If you learn this, you will always have a job. No matter what happens, you can always fall back on dental assisting. There is always going to be a need for you." So, as I headed into college, I thought, "OK, dental assisting will be my backup." Dentistry wasn't my goal. I wanted to go into medicine, and I completed four years of premed. But when it came time to take the MCAT, I kept thinking about dentistry, and I had this intuition that I should take the DAT, too, and see which one I did better on. But the tests were being held on the exact same day; I had to make a decision. I chose to take the DAT, and I didn't look back. In the end, it turned out to be the right decision.

In dental school, we were assigned patients. We treated some children, but mostly we treated adults. I found myself starting to incorporate with my adult patients what I had seen my stepdad do with his patients. I would just listen. I would ask questions about their lives and what they were interested in. I would just get people talking, and like my stepfather, I would tune out the entire world and make that one patient my entire focus.

I continued connecting this way with my patients in my practices. When I was about ten years out of school, and my ex-husband and I were still in practice together and sharing patients, I noticed that more and more women requested to see me personally. When I finally opened my own practice, which is about fifteen miles from my previous one and the community that knew me, right out of the box, I started seeing more adult patients.

Again, it is unusual for an orthodontist to have such a high adult patient caseload, but they kept seeking me out. Yes, I'm a talented orthodontist, and I will give you an amazing smile, but I think adults seek me out for the intangibles. It's how they feel when they are in my practice and how they feel after they leave. I want them to feel good, to feel heard and cared about. I want this especially for the women we treat. As women, we often put the other people in our lives first. Some of us are just wired that way, some of us are trained that way, and some of us just feel guilty if we don't. We are the caretakers in our worlds, and with that comes so many responsibilities. It's important to me to provide an environment where women can truly be cared for and be able to recharge in an environment that nurtures their inner smiles as my team and I work to brighten their outer smiles. I don't just want to look at their teeth; I want to look at the whole person and hear that whole person. My perspective as an orthodontist is unique because I know the demands that are on women; I live with those same demands.

> It's important to me to provide an environment where women can truly be cared for and be able to recharge in an environment that nurtures their inner smiles as my team and I work to brighten their outer smiles.

Several years ago, I knew I had to make a major life shift to find my joy, to reignite my inner smile, and return to my true path. And you know what I learned? If you have to upend a lot of things to get to that point, it's OK. Through this process, I have done a lot of work on myself—work that required me to address a lot of challenges in my life and forced me to focus on what I'm about and who I am as a mom, as an orthodontist, as a professional, as a friend, as a wife, and also as an ex-wife. It was incredibly difficult for me. What I've learned and what I've worked through have helped me realize the importance of listening to my inner voice and trusting it.

Through my story, I want people, especially women, to know that it's OK to be who you are, even if that means going against social conventions or ruffling someone's feathers. It's so important to listen to and trust your inner voice—that's how you will find the path that you're meant to be on. In the end, when you listen to your inner voice and take action, you are going to be a better mom, partner, professional—a better you.

Know that whoever you are, it's OK to own it.

CHAPTER 1

CHAPTER 1

THE MAGIC OF ORTHODONTICS

If you see someone without a smile, give them one of yours.
—*DOLLY PARTON*

My daily joy comes from the partnerships I develop with my patients. My practice is about looking at the whole person and hearing the whole person—asking what do they want and what's going on in their lives. My team and I take the time to get to know our patients and genuinely connect with them from the first point of contact. This is an important part of the process from the beginning. When I do initial consultations, I have to make sure that the treatment I recommend works for that patient's teeth but also works for the individual, their lifestyle, and their family.

Adults can be complicated, and it's more than just their teeth that we need to address. We try to help them figure out what's out of balance in either their health or their life, and how that contributes to what's going on with their teeth or their jaws. Our patients talk with my staff and me about what's going on in their lives, whether it's about something that happened at work or with their kids or their spouse. My practice is a place where people can feel comfortable and safe just talking and feeling heard and cared for. *Sanctuary* is the term for this type of environment, and it is one that I strive to create in all aspects of my life.

I've had some of the women who come into my office go back out into the reception area after their appointments, and they sit for a while and read; they don't want to leave. They tell us, "It's peaceful here. I have some time; I'm just going to hang out a little bit." Knowing they feel that way about my office, that they feel so comfortable in this space, means everything to me.

I know how important that kind of space to just be yourself is. I know that sometimes our outer smiles belie our inner smiles, and I know how challenging that can be. I know because I have experienced it as a child and as an adult. Life moves so quickly, and we get caught up in it. Several years ago, I found myself at that point. Life was rushing in, and I started asking myself, "Is this really the life I want? Where am I? How did I get here?"

Things just built up and built up, and then I just had a complete implosion when I decided I couldn't do it anymore. I woke up and knew I had to make some terribly difficult decisions that I didn't want to make, because it meant a divorce and leaving the practice that I had built up for so long, and that I loved so much. But I realized that somewhere along the way, I stopped listening to my inner voice, and I knew that these significant changes had to happen for me to get back on my true path and reignite my own inner smile.

ALWAYS LEAVING

When I was one year old, my father moved out of our home when my parents divorced. Soon afterward, my mother and I moved in with my grandparents and my sixteen-year-old uncle in St. Louis. My grandfather became my father figure, but as a river boat pilot on the Mississippi River, he was absent a lot. Two years later, my beloved uncle went off to college at the University of Missouri. The following year, my mother, as a single mom trying to better herself so she could support me, applied for and was accepted into a government program that enabled her to obtain her master's degree at a very low cost. But the program was at the University of North Carolina, so when I was three years old, my mother left me with my grandparents for a year to pursue her master's.

A sense of abandonment was something I experienced a lot in the first years of my life, which deeply affected me, because I thought, as any child would, that it was my fault. I think my having experienced significant people leaving me is why, even at the young ages of four and five, I always wanted to be around people, especially other children. I would enjoy the company of my neighborhood friends so much that when it was time to go home, I would beg them to promise me that we would play again tomorrow. I loved the connection with these friends, and I was always worried that I wouldn't see them again.

My grandmother was my one constant in my early years, and she was amazing; she became my anchor. Even so, the separation of starting school was difficult for me. And because I was familiar with people leaving me, when I was at school, I would worry that everyone would be gone when I returned home. It was very difficult for me, and as a result, I dreaded school.

But I also found things to love about school. I loved being around the other students. I did everything I could to connect with them, and I loved learning. As my grandmother was my anchor at home, my best friend, Linda, was my anchor at school. Linda was my first friend; we've known each other since we were three. Linda has always been a very strong, solid person and a solid friend, and fortunately, we were in the same kindergarten class.

Kindergarten is when testing begins to see what reading level you are at, and my testing revealed that I was reading at a third or fourth grade level. This meant that when it was reading time, a tutor would come down and take me out of the room, away from my friends, to keep me moving ahead. This was devastating for me, because all I wanted to do was fit in. I just wanted to be a part of everybody, and I didn't want anyone to think of me as different.

Being taken out of my classroom for reading was difficult for me, and it continued through the next couple of years. In third grade, when they put me in the high-level group, I knew I did not want to be there. I didn't like the teacher, and I didn't like kids in the class.

> **Your ability may be at a certain point, but that doesn't mean that's the point where you're happiest.**

Back then I couldn't clearly articulate what it was I wanted or why; I just knew the high-level group did not feel right to me. And Linda was in the second-level group, and I didn't like being separated from her. Looking back, at the age of eight, I was already listening to my inner voice without realizing what it was. At that age, my inner voice spoke through crying. I cried a lot and wouldn't want to go to school because I was so upset.

Eventually, I was allowed to move into the second-level group to be with Linda. And you know what? It turned out great. I was happier there. Sometimes societal expectations push you in one direction, but maybe that doesn't match with who you are. Your ability may be at a certain point, but that doesn't mean that's the point where you're happiest. I was grateful to have remained with my friends in third grade, because unbeknownst to me, I would be changing schools the following year.

At the end of my third grade, my mom remarried, which meant I had to move to a different school. That was devastating for me. Not only was it a much smaller school (25 students in an entire grade, as opposed to 250 per grade at my previous school,) but it also was a Catholic school, and I was not Catholic. We had to wear uniforms, and there was no gym, no cafeteria, no playground.

DROPPING THE REINS

My mom's marriage also included us moving out to a horse farm about twenty miles south of St. Louis. No longer being in a neighborhood felt very isolating for me. Linda was no longer next door, and I had no friends down the street. We were in the middle of nowhere. Linda would come out and stay with me for a weekend, or I'd spend time at her house, but it was lonely on the farm. Between my struggle switching schools and being so far from my friends, I was sad, and I continued to cry a lot.

My new stepfather was our dentist. He was beloved by the community. He was very charismatic, the kind of person whose energy fills a room. Initially, I think he tried to make things as normal as possible, but within a year or two, his struggles with alcohol addiction became apparent. During the week, we were still a typical family. We'd eat dinner together and have a normal routine, but then on weekends, he began drinking and partying. Often, my mom would leave him wherever they had gone out. If they went to the racetrack to watch our horses run, she would leave him there after he drank for a while, and someone would drive him home much later.

Many times, I'd hear him come in at three or four o'clock in the morning, yelling and screaming and wanting to keep the party going. It was very scary for me to see this other person who was so different from the stepdad I knew at his dental office and at home during the week. As I got older, I understood more about what was happening, but it was still uncomfortable, because he was so unpredictable when he was drinking.

My environment felt unstable again, and I threw myself into my schoolwork. It provided me a sense of control, and it was so important to me to do well. I also started riding horses. I was a natural at it, and I loved it. Learning to ride filled a void for me. We had horses at our farm, but I trained with different stables around the area. Two of the stables were high profile on the national circuit, and the people I rode with were the elite of St. Louis. Their parents had lots of money, and they attended the expensive private schools in St. Louis. I was embarrassed about where I lived out in the country and therefore never had any of my riding friends over to my house. Nevertheless, my strong desire to connect with people enabled me to blend in and make friends.

Again, I found myself hiding who I really was. As I reflect back, a theme emerges of me being embarrassed about what my life is like and trying to pretend that my life is something different than it is.

I was a very good rider—I immersed myself in the riding world when I was not studying and doing my schoolwork. It was highly competitive. I rode in the circuit traveling all over this half of the country. I practiced four days a week, two to three hours a day after school. My stepdad was the type of person who really instilled the mindset that "if you're not first, you're last," just like in the movie *Talladega Nights*. I was told and taught the lesson: "We don't compete to compete; we compete to win and dominate." And I did do well; I was nationally ranked. Whenever I won, I felt like my stepdad wanted to own my successes; he did this with his other children's successes, too, even when we did well in school. He was proud, of course, but it went well beyond that. It was like he saw our successes as a reflection of him.

When I started high school, I was burned out on riding, and I wanted to have a social life. I had been riding competitively for five years, and after I won state championships in two separate divisions, I was exhausted, and I wanted to take a year off from competing. As it turned out, I never went back. I hit my peak at thirteen; I was done by fourteen. That was all there was to it. I realized I had lost the joy of riding that had been there in the early days. It had turned into a big competition with everyone always pushing for the wins, so I just dropped the reins, so to speak. I was done.

Dropping the reins is part of an actual exercise riders practice. You tie the reins in a knot and lay them on the horse's neck and then go down lines of jumps without holding the reins, your arms straight out, controlling the horse with only your legs. This exercise develops your core and your balance and trust in working with the horse through your body and your legs. It's exhilarating and scary, but when you do it, it's amazing.

> **At some point, you just have to drop the reins and let the Universe do what it's going to do.**

In life, we often find ourselves trying so hard to control our circumstances or trying to make sure everything's okay all the time, and it just doesn't work. It will work for a while, but it is exhausting and draining, and at some point, you just have to drop the reins and let the Universe do what it's going to do. You just have to trust you're making the right decision. That's a metaphor I often think about and use in my life. I need to just drop the reins and trust.

Not only did I stop riding at the beginning of high school, but that is also when my stepdad moved out. My mother and stepfather did not end the marriage at that time; they separated physically, but we would still spend time as a family on some weekends and vacations. That was weird for me. Again I found myself feeling like I was different, not "normal," and I just wanted to blend in and belong with my peers, so I tried to hide my real family life from people. I just didn't talk about my family, not even to my friends. Linda knew and had experienced much of it with me, but we did not talk about it. I didn't know how to explain it, and I was embarrassed about it. I went to a Catholic high school out in the country where everyone was very conventional. At that time, in the '80s, few parents of classmates were divorced, let alone remarried and then separated.

It was a disruptive and challenging home life, and I wanted to hide and avoid it as much as possible. During high school, I was out with my friends a lot. I would spend time at their houses instead of mine. I just tried to be as "normal" as I could and tried to have some control in other aspects of my life, and that meant when I wasn't with my friends, I was studying. My studying was probably beyond normal. I was a chronic overachiever, but I could control that, and that control gave me comfort.

DECIDING ON DENTISTRY

In May of 1982, I turned sixteen, and my social life was flourishing. Several of my friends had turned sixteen at the beginning of the school year, so they already had their driver's licenses, and we would pile into cars, go out, and just have fun. I was so excited to turn sixteen and get my license. I envisioned that the whole summer would be going to every pool party with my girlfriends, partying all day, hanging out, but my parents had other ideas. I was told, "You're going to work at the office," and that's how I spent my summer, working at my stepfather's dental practice.

When I started, I really resisted. I did not want to go. Being there pushed the boundaries of my comfort level; I was sixteen and wondering why I would want to put my hands in people's mouths. I wasn't sure I could even do it. Luckily, I began working at the front desk, filing charts, answering phones, and scheduling while I eased into clinic work.

Later in the summer, I started doing simple assisting like suctioning. My stepdad's assistants were wonderful, and they did a great job training me. Being on the clinical side, I saw my stepdad through a different set of eyes. To see the way he interacted with his patients, no matter who they were, was amazing. I've never seen a dentist before or since who has that sort of relationship with their patients. Whether they were six or sixty, he'd take their hands, and he'd ask, "What's going on? How are you doing today?" He genuinely cared about the answer, and it lit people up. I really was amazed.

Seeing this side of him brought some resentment on my part. I wondered how he could be so great with his patients and then be so different in his family life when there was alcohol involved. This was a time when I could see him truly as he was and how he made people feel without any substance, without any alcohol. It was really, really astounding.

The following summer I did a higher level of assisting. I was trained to do almost everything with him that all his main assistants would do, whether it was helping with extractions or making a temporary crown. It took a while for me to shake off the resentment and warm up to being there, but I eventually accepted that when we were at work, I needed to put everything else aside. Here he was Dr. West and not Dad. At that point, I was able to observe and learn what I could from him during my summers in high school.

In college I studied premed. I was always going to be a doctor. I can remember thinking as early as four or five, that I wanted to be a doctor. In the '70s most girls were told to be secretaries, nurses, or teachers. My grandmother used to say, "You can do anything you want if you put your mind to it." And my mother was a strong role model for me professionally. She always said, "You always have to be able to provide for yourself. You can never depend on anyone else to support you. You have to do it for yourself." So when I was a little girl, there was no doubt in my mind that I could be whatever I wanted.

As the deadline for me to take the MCATs drew closer, I began thinking about my experience with my stepdad in his practice, and about how my favorite uncle is a dentist, and that I had loved going to my orthodontist when I was younger. I began to wonder, "Would dentistry be such a bad thing? I could be my own boss. I could do a lot of things." My biggest concern was that I did not want to end up working with my stepdad in his practice—I wanted to have my own path, my own unique career independent of my stepdad.

I decided I was going to let the Universe decide; I would take the MCAT for medical school and the DAT for dental school. I would prepare for both, and whichever one I did better on, that was going to be my answer. As it turned out, the Universe would not decide my fate after all. The MCAT and DAT were held on the exact same day. They were offered one time in April. That's it. So I had to make my decision.

After a lot of meditating, I knew I had to listen to my inner voice of where I needed to go. I chose the DATs, and I rocked them. Schools were rolling out the red carpet for me. I chose Northwestern University Dental School in Chicago, and I graduated first in my DDS class, and then I received my MS in orthodontics from the University of Michigan, which remains number one in the world in dental school rankings.

WHY CHOOSE ORTHODONTICS?

When I was entering my third year of dental school, I had thought that I was going to be an oral surgeon. One of my mentors in dental school, Dr. Donald Hoffman, arranged for me to attend an oral surgery program and participate in a special externship at a St. Louis hospital between my third and fourth years of dental school. I was enthralled with oral surgery from day one; I loved being in the hospital setting with both ER and scheduled cases. I thrived in the environment, and becoming an oral surgeon would satisfy my previous desire to go to medical school.

The externship ended all too quickly, and I drove back to Chicago. That drive provided me a lot of quiet time to reflect on where I was going and what I wanted. I had to admit that oral surgery was exciting and seductive, but would that be enough to sustain me long term? I had this sense that a path of oral surgery meant that there wouldn't be room left in my life for anything else. Over the next several months, I was in an internal tug-of-war between wanting to be an oral surgeon and wanting to also have a personal life, to be a wife and a mother.

In the end, it was Dr. Hoffman who provided me the insight I was seeking. He had no doubt about my ability to be an outstanding oral surgeon, but he said that knowing me and who I am and what I wanted to have in life, he felt I should seriously consider the orthodontic specialty. That's when I embraced the idea of living my life as an orthodontist.

CHAPTER 2

THERE IS NO SUCH THING AS "JUST SMILING"

When you're smiling, the whole world smiles with you.
—LOUIS ARMSTRONG

Sharing and receiving smiles have the power to lift our spirits, shift the mood of a room, and positively impact our outlook. I remember a smile moment from when I was in college, and I was traveling around visiting dental schools. I was out to dinner in Boston with a friend of mine, and we had hopped up to the bar and were chatting away. The bartender walked by and said that he would be right with us. I smiled at him and told him that sounded great. That simple gesture stopped him in his tracks, and he said, "You have such a nice smile. It makes me happy." Thirty years later, that simple yet powerful exchange is still ingrained in my memory. This person's evening was positively altered just because I smiled at him, and it made me feel good too.

I have also benefited from the smiles I have received. Dental school was incredibly difficult. It is a year-round schedule with only four weeks of break throughout the year, so you feel wrung out and exhausted most of the time. During the most trying times, it was my good friend Jim's smile that buoyed my spirits and got me through. I can remember moments of feeling down, and Jim would say something funny and then flash me his bright smile. It was contagious, and all I could do was return the smile, and it lifted the clouds away for me. Jim was truly a master at shifting the mood of everyone around him with his genuine smile.

There are times for everyone when smiling can be challenging. Perhaps they are self-conscious of how their teeth look, or they are experiencing life struggles that create sadness and stress. I know that when I'm having a stressful day or experiencing a challenging time, I consciously try to smile my way out of it, and honestly, it does seem to help. I recently read about a 114-year-old man in Japan who was asked to reveal his secret to longevity. His answer? "Smiling." That's it, just one word: smiling.

Seems too simple, right? But there is research to back up his answer. According to Ron Gutman in his TEDTalk "The Hidden Power of Smiling," smiling influences many aspects of our lives, including longevity:[1]

> My own aha! moment on just how impactful smiling can
> be, came from a 2010 Wayne State University research project
> that looked into pre-1950s baseball cards of Major League
> players. The researchers found that the span of a player's smile
> could actually predict the span of his life. Players who didn't

---

1   Ron Gutman, "The Hidden Power of Smiling," filmed
    March 2011. TED video, 7:11, https://www.ted.com/talks/
    ron_gutman_the_hidden_power_of_smiling?language=en.

smile in their pictures lived an average of only 72.9 years, where
players with beaming smiles lived an average of almost 80 years.

I know a smile can't cure everything. There are circumstances of grief, mental illness, and physical health issues that significantly impact our ability to smile. But even in those instances, pushing ourselves to smile can have a positive impact. In Gutman's TED Talk, he went on to explain some of the science behind our smiles:[2]

> *In a German study related to Darwin's facial feedback*
> *response theory, researchers used fMRI imaging to measure*
> *brain activity before and after injecting Botox to suppress*
> *smiling muscles. The finding supported Darwin's theory by*
> *showing that facial feedback modifies the neural processing*
> *of emotional content in the brain in a way that helps us feel*
> *better when we smile. Smiling stimulates our brain reward*
> *mechanism in a way that even chocolate—a well-regarded*
> *pleasure inducer—cannot match.*
>
> *British researchers found that one smile can generate the*
> *same level of brain stimulation as up to 2,000 bars of chocolate.*
> *And unlike lots of chocolate, lots of smiling can actually make*
> *you healthier. Smiling can help reduce the level of stress-enhanc-*
> *ing hormones like cortisol, adrenaline and dopamine, increase*
> *the level of mood-enhancing hormones like endorphins, and*
> *reduce overall blood pressure.*

I notice that if I consciously smile at someone or take a moment when I'm talking with a patient to just add a smile, it immediately shifts my attitude and focus. It pulls me out of any negative energy that I might be carrying. It's incredibly powerful.

---

2   Ibid.

If I am with a new patient who is feeling anxious, and I greet them with a smile, I can almost see their anxiety wash away. If you smile at yourself in the mirror, or just think of something funny that makes you smile, it really can change your whole brain chemistry. Smiling can change your whole attitude and connect you back with yourself and other people.

> **Smiling can change your whole attitude and connect you back with yourself and other people.**

BE MY GUEST

My practice is built around making people smile—not just orthodontically, but also by how we engage with our patients. I crafted the whole practice based on human connection. What that means is truly listening and meeting each patient where they are in that moment. When we ask our patients how they are doing, they know that we are not asking just about their teeth; we are asking about their whole person.

We have parents and families who have different challenges in their personal lives, and we try to recognize that. It's always been important to me to check in with people and make sure they are OK. When a patient comes in and they're having a rough day, we do our best to let them know that we care. What that means is different for each person; sometimes that's a smile, sometimes that's space. I have two teenagers at home, and I understand that sometimes the best thing you can do for a person is to not do anything, and just be respectful of their space and let them know that you're there if they need you. I'm fortunate to have an amazing staff who recognizes these important subtleties.

Our patients, at different stages in their orthodontic process, spend a lot of time with each of my staff, so it's incredibly important that we are all in sync and looking in the same direction in regard to how we treat people. When our patients walk in our door, they are greeted by their name and with a smile. Greeting everyone this way says to me, *Welcome to my home*. And that is exactly how I want our patients to feel—like they are a guest in my home. We carry this through to every part of the practice and through every interaction they have with any team member.

A POSITIVE INFLUENCE

As my journey to dentistry was an evolution, so, too, was my journey to being a more thoughtful and compassionate practitioner. Because there have been many challenges in my life, I had to learn to rein in my thoughts of negativity and overthinking the actions of others. Growing up, I always took things so personally, and if something wasn't right or someone was unhappy, I would worry that it was my fault and that I needed to fix it. I really had to work hard on shifting my whole mindset, stepping back, and seeing the situation for what it was … which, as it turns out, generally had nothing to do with me.

Looking at my practice and the effort we put into making patients feel like guests—and the effort I've put into shifting my mindset from one of insecurity to confidence and positivity—I can't help but appreciate the influence that Dr. Jim McNamara had in that outcome. Jim was my thesis advisor; he invited me into his practice when I first graduated, and he is my son's godfather. Jim has been influential in many aspects of my life—how I practice orthodontics, how I relate to others, and how I treat my patients. They are guests—I learned that from him.

When I first joined his practice, we would share patients. That meant when he was gone, I would see his patients in order to eliminate any interruption in their treatment plan. It was challenging for me as a new graduate to treat patients who were accustomed to being seen by an orthodontist with over twenty years of experience. Jim recognized this and took me aside. He said, "Look, there are going to be a variety of parents and patients, some more challenging than others … and, well, they're all used to me. You cannot take it personally when they ask, 'What would Dr. McNamara do?' or 'Where is Dr. McNamara?' or 'I want to see Dr. McNamara.' Do not worry about that. Don't take that to heart. That doesn't matter. Because you will grow and develop, so don't let that derail you."

And he was right: I did continue to grow and develop under his guidance. Jim was a well-respected lecturer, author, and educator, and all of those qualities benefited me as a new orthodontist. As an educator, Jim was always willing to teach—what we called calibrating. He would call me over to take a look at what he was doing for a patient that had an unusual or complicated issue, and he would explain why he was doing what he was doing and ask if I had any questions. As a well-respected authority in orthodontics, Jim often treated some of the most complex and challenging cases, such as individuals with cleft palates and craniofacial defects, all of which I was fortunate to observe and learn from.

Jim's kind and generous guidance over the years helped me tremendously in the development of my abilities as an orthodontist, both the artistic and technical aspects, as well as my journey to become more compassionate about what other people's journeys are. Jim is a positive person. I've never heard him, in all my years of knowing him, say anything negative about another person, which is incredible. I have never heard him complain about anything. If there's a problem, his attitude is, "We'll deal with it." That's quite an elevated level for a person to aspire to, but providing my patients the positive, kind, and compassionate connections that Jim modeled for me is what I aspire to do every day. And to do be able to do it with a smile is the greatest gift of all.

CHAPTER 3

YOUR OUTER SMILE

A smile is a curve that sets everything straight.
—PHYLLIS DILLER

When you smile at yourself in the mirror, does the image please you? Are your teeth straight, bright, and pleasingly proportioned? Do they physically feel good, strong, and healthy, not making speaking or eating awkward for you, not chipped, broken, or discolored?

The first time I meet with a new patient, I don't assume anything. I do the initial examination and take photographs and then we meet, and I listen. I learned early on that what I see from an orthodontic perspective may not be a concern for that individual, so my role is to listen and ask questions based on the information they are providing.

I once treated an older gentleman when I was in dental school who had to get a set of dentures. He'd gotten a crown on one of his front teeth years ago that was gold, so he brought in the gold crown and wanted me to put it in the denture because that was really important to him. People want different things, and I learned that what my idea of what will make a patient happy—a beautiful, perfect denture with no gold crowns, for example—maybe isn't what the patient wants. This gentleman wanted a gold tooth in the front. When he smiled, he wanted some gold showing, and that made him the happiest person in the world. People have their own ideas of what they want, and it's important to honor and respect that.

That said, most people do not come in saying, "OK, time to get my smile on; let's do this." They may not know what they want, because they don't know what options they have and how many possibilities there are. They are more likely to come in and tell me what they don't like about how their teeth or smile look and ask if I can help. Once I start to show patients what we can do for them, I see this spark of hope.

Now, with innovative technology, we can show what the outcome of potential treatment will look like through visual simulation. Especially for our adults, this creates so much excitement and optimism when they realize that they can be happy with their teeth, their smiles, and the overall aesthetics of their faces. It opens a new world for them, and from there we start to talk more about quality of life. Are they having any jaw joint problems, facial pain, or other issues? That's when we can have a more holistic dialogue and talk about potential root causes of these issues and concerns. Sometimes that cause may be stress, and we will offer them stress management ideas.

Many adults that we see have spent years with physical or visual discomfort with their jaws, teeth, or smiles, so when they come to us, they are ready to consider a change. But even though they are emotionally ready, it's challenging for adults to commit because they have busy, full lives, and they have to consider how the time commitment to orthodontics will impact everything else they have going on. That's just the reality. What I tell patients—and I truly believe this—is that time is going to move forward, regardless of whether they do the treatment or not. They're still going to be working, parenting, doing whatever they are doing, and they'll reach a point in the hustle and bustle of their life when their treatment could have already been completed. There will never be a time that taking care of their mouth, their teeth, or their smiles will fit perfectly into their lives, but it's still important to take care of themselves. I tell them to let me handle it. I'll take care of their teeth while they take care of their life.

I have so many patients who say after treatment, "I wish I did this sooner." I have one patient in her fifties who, when she came to us, had suffered for years with jaw and facial pain. The pain was making her miserable; it was like a dark cloud constantly hanging over her. We started her Invisalign treatment, and when she came back ten weeks later for her first follow-up, she had already experienced a dramatic difference. She came in and said, "I can't believe it; I haven't felt this good in years! Why did I wait so long?" As her treatment has progressed, we've seen an incredible change in her whole aura. She has a new buoyancy about her; she's not exhausted anymore, because she is no longer in constant pain. Now she has a reason to truly smile.

> **Whether we are helping to relieve chronic pain or building confidence in someone's smile, we are building relationships with our patients, and we are lucky enough to be invited into their lives during the time that they are with us.**

And that's what it is all about: bringing out inner and outer smiles. Whether we are helping to relieve chronic pain or building confidence in someone's smile, we are building relationships with our patients, and we are lucky enough to be invited into their lives during the time that they are with us. I've had expectant parents who are so excited to finish their treatment in time for the arrival of their babies. I had one mom tell me, "I want to introduce myself to my child with my beautiful smile." It's such an honor for me to be able to share parts of my patients' journeys with them. Creating space for those connections is intentional. I chose to craft a smaller practice so I could be more involved with my patients. In the larger practice that I used to own, my face time with patients was so fleeting, and it all became a blur. My practice now is a labor of love and connection.

WHY SEVEN IS A MAGIC AGE

The American Association of Orthodontists recommends that children be screened by an orthodontist at age seven. The benchmark of seven was established because by that age, the top and bottom front permanent teeth have come in, as well as the first permanent molars. Our goal with young kids is to work with their growth. If they come in at a young age for a screening, we are able to get a read on how their jaws are growing—are they growing proportionally, is there a tooth-crowding issue, is there an underlying muscular or functional imbalance? It's beneficial to identify issues with their jaws and teeth early, because we don't want to later be paddling upstream against a growth-pattern issue—we want to work with them while they're growing. That's the optimal time to create more space and make structural adjustments to prevent having to extract any permanent teeth later and to try to prevent avoidable dental work as an adult.

I approach our young patients with the same open inquiry as I do our adult patients. A parent will provide me the initial overview, but then I start interacting with the child right away, no matter how old they are. I ask them things like, "Is there anything about your teeth that you don't like? Is there anything that hurts when you chew food?" I'm listening and watching for their speech pattern. I'm assessing a lot of things when I'm asking questions and getting them to talk about themselves without them even realizing it. When they start sharing with me, that's when I might be able to identify an issue that we can fix that might make it easier for them to take care of their teeth, to swallow or speak or chew, or eliminate some pain or discomfort.

The varying degrees of self-confidence and perceptions are no different with children than they are with adults. We have kids who are embarrassed if their teeth are the slightest shade off white. I think that is a result of the photoshopped smiles we see everywhere. But it's on their mind, so we talk about it. Then we have the kids who come in whose teeth are everywhere; they're just a mash-up. And I'll ask them if there is anything they don't like about their teeth, and they'll smile and say, "Nope!" They just aren't concerned about how their teeth look at that point, and like with adults, we listen and meet them where they're at. If there is a structural issue that needs to be addressed, then we'll have that conversation with the parent.

I've had kids come in who have impaired speech because of a structural problem. Over time, we'll correct it, and suddenly their transformation is like night and day. Their speech has changed. They're not having to go to speech therapy anymore. That makes a world of difference for that child. Being able to identify and correct something as significant as a speech sound disorder for a child is huge. Untreated, that structural issue could have caused other dental challenges in addition to prolonging the psychological toll a speech disorder can take on a child. Life-changing impacts like this are what drive the recommendation for orthodontic screening at the age of seven.

BRIDGING PARTNERSHIPS

Many of our patients are referred to us by their dentists. There are some dentists who will send every child over at the age of seven for a screening. Other dentists might be more in tune with orthodontic treatments, and they are able to recognize what I would recognize. In those cases, they will monitor the child until they know it's time for orthodontic work to begin, and then they will refer them over.

> **One of the best things you can do for your oral health is to have a primary dentist.**

Whenever a patient is referred to us, or if they come to us on their own, I'll reach out to their dentist and let them know that I saw their patient and what my evaluation is and ask them if they have any questions. It's important to have strong relationships with my patients' dentists; I always let the dentists know that my practice is here to support both them and our mutual patients as we care for them.

One of the best things you can do for your oral health is to have a primary dentist. I tell my patients that their dentist is their home base, and we are just part of the team that's supporting their dentist's long-term care. Our patients are with us temporarily, maybe one or two or three years, kids a little longer. Ultimately, I "graduate" them from my practice, and their primary dentist will continue to take care of them, and I can get called in from the sidelines if I'm needed.

It's your dentist who is also going to care for your gum health, which is critical to your overall health. There are strong correlations between gum disease and diabetes, heart disease, stroke, and other significant health issues. It's critical that you keep your gums healthy, so that you're not contributing to other health issues. More detailed information is on the American Academy of Periodontology website, perio.org. Your dentist is also going to be the first to notice a cavity, an abscess, or any other concern with your mouth that, if left untreated, could be serious. So your dentist, along with daily flossing and brushing, is your first line of defense for good oral health. Regular care is critical. If you let something go too long, and your gum or dental health deteriorates, it's going to take longer to correct—if it can still be fully corrected. Think of it like a parallel in your life journey: the longer you're on the wrong path, the harder it is to get onto your right path.

SMILING IS CONTAGIOUS

Over the past twenty-five years of practice, I have had the honor of giving the gift of a smile to thousands of people. I know firsthand how contagious they are. I have seen it in the countless smiles I have received and given—and you know what? It never gets old. A smile always makes everything new again. As renowned motivational speaker Brian Tracy shared, "When you smile at another person, the physical action releases endorphins in your brain. Endorphins are called nature's 'happy drug.' They make you feel happy and raise your self-esteem. When you smile, you feel and act in a more personable way to everyone around and exude a feeling of positive attitude."[3]

Got a smile? Go ahead and share it!

---

3   Brian Tracy, "How a Smile can Affect Self-Esteem: Building Healthy Relationships with a Positive Attitude," Brian Tracy International, February 11, 2016.

CHAPTER 4

FEELING GOOD FROM THE INSIDE OUT

Count your life by smiles, not tears. A dream
you dream alone is only a dream.
—*JOHN LENNON*

By the time I graduated dental school and completed my orthodontic residency, I had so much knowledge. I had eleven years of schooling and training behind me, and I was ready to jump in. But it wasn't until I did jump in that I realized how little I knew about the practical, real-life aspects of practicing orthodontics. Fortunately, I had key role models to teach me the ropes of patient treatment and practice management.

Right out of school, I was off and running in several different directions. I was teaching, and I was practicing with Dr. Jim McNamara and with Dr. David Kott—three different experiences that provided their own unique wisdoms that I would carry throughout my career.

TEACHING

I had recently completed my orthodontic residency and was back on campus one day when I popped in to say hi to my former chairman, Dr. Lysle Johnston, head of the Department of Orthodontics and Pediatric Dentistry. It turns out he had just gotten off the phone with an instructor who had given notice that they were leaving, and he offered me their now-open teaching opportunity. I was so fortunate to be there at the right moment, and for twenty-four years, I taught the Development of Occlusion and Interceptive Orthodontics course at the University of Michigan.

The course focuses on early treatment of developing dentition, primarily with kids between the ages of seven and twelve. It encompasses facial growth, tooth eruption, malocclusion, and other developmental issues, examining how and when you can intercept specific problems, correct them as needed, and prevent further damage down the road. I lectured to first-year orthodontic residents fresh out of dental school who usually came in with little or no previous orthodontic knowledge. That they came with a clean slate was great, because my class would teach them the fundamentals upon which to build their knowledge.

Having taught the course for so many years, I was always reviewing the content to make sure I was keeping it fresh. One thing I liked to do is include real-world examples. I remember one session when I lectured on the practical aspects of case management and the family finances of a patient. In dental school and in orthodontic residency, patients are prescreened and handed over or assigned to the students when the patient is ready for treatment. As a student, you are mostly charged with learning and performing hands-on dental and orthodontic work with little involvement in the diagnosis and treatment planning of a case. In the real world, when a patient comes into your office, they need to be thoroughly evaluated and assessed for treatment. It's possible that treatment won't happen for a few months or maybe a couple of years, and the orthodontist is tasked with monitoring the patient's growth and development in the interim.

The other part of that equation is talking with the family about when they will be financially ready to do x, y, and z treatment. It is a critical component of practice management and one you don't tend think of as an orthodontic resident. I tried to share the full picture of patient treatment with my students. For example, if someone asks me when their child will be ready to start treatment so they can create a savings plan to pay for it, and I answer twelve months but the child actually becomes ready in six, I have just created a possible financial hardship for the family. An orthodontist can't plan it perfectly, but they must be as accurate as possible. Understanding normal growth, eruption, and development is critical—if you don't know what is normal, you cannot know what is abnormal. After one of the lectures in which I discussed this topic in detail, I had a student come up to me and ask, "Do you have any tips on how to get bands (braces) on the upper back second molars?"

That was a reality check for me! These students are still trying to get their bearings and figure out the mechanics of putting braces on and are far from the nuances of patient finances and how to properly manage a practice at this stage of their education. I still included real-world experience in my lectures, but this was one of those moments that reminded me to meet the students where they are in their journey and to remember all the things they may have going on in their life in addition to the intensity of orthodontic training.

All the years of teaching have kept me connected to younger people in a way that I would have missed otherwise. When I first started teaching, I was only a year or two older than my students. Now that I have two decades of experience, I am often also a mentor to my students and make myself available to walk them through opening a practice, building a practice, and the hands-on business aspects after they have graduated and are ready to strike out on their own.

GETTING DOWN TO BUSINESS

Out of My Comfort Zone

As I shared in chapter 2, Dr. McNamara welcomed me into his practice straight out of my orthodontic residency and taught me orthodontics on so many levels. He also taught me aspects of the business that I didn't even know existed. What they don't tell you in dental school or orthodontic residency is that when you join a practice, one of the hats you inevitably wear is that of marketer. Often the expectation is that each orthodontist contributes new patients to the practice; you have to bring in new referrals to cover your salary and keep the practice growing.

> What they don't tell you in dental school or orthodontic residency is that when you join a practice, one of the hats you inevitably wear is that of marketer.

True to form, I had a job to do, and I was going to do it to the best of my ability, so I hit the ground running. Marketing back then was primarily going to dental offices, introducing yourself to the dentist, hopefully scheduling a lunch, and if you were really good at it, working in a round of golf with as many of them as possible. This type of forced engagement was way out of my comfort zone.

My first go, I was given the dental directory of the Ann Arbor area and told, "The dentists highlighted are the ones already referring to us; now go see everyone else." It was intimidating to reach out to these dentists for a number of reasons, but especially because I had no idea why they weren't referring to us; was it just because they already had other partnerships, or had there been some type of negative incident? It was my job to bridge the gap with any of the dentists who weren't already referring to Dr. McNamara.

I was young and new, and most of the dentists that I needed to reach out to were much older than me and entrenched in the good ol' boys' club. Many times they were busy with patients and wouldn't even take a minute to see me. Often they'd ask me to just leave a business card or referral pad, and if I was lucky, all I would have time to get in is, "I just wanted to say hi, put a face with a name. I look forward to working with you. Hope we can work together."

There was one dentist, Dr. Tom Slade, who still stands out in my mind today for his kindness. His was one of the many offices I walked into hoping to build a rapport. I remember being terrified to go in there, and he turned out to be this giant-sized former football player; his presence alone was intimidating, and he was incredibly busy. But he stopped and made the time to see me, and we started talking, and he made me feel so comfortable—it was such a welcomed surprise. Dr. Slade became one of our biggest referrals over the years. It just takes one positive interaction like that to boost your confidence.

Although the whole marketing requirement made me uncomfortable, it was good for me to be pushed out of my comfort zone and learn how to do it, because it prepared me for when I bought my first practice and didn't know any dentists in the area. I was grateful that I knew how to build those partnerships.

Practice Management

Shortly after graduating, in addition to practicing in Dr. McNamara's practice, I joined Dr. David Kott's practice. Dr. Kott always hired a recent Michigan orthodontic graduate. I spent two years there working two days a week just putting braces on and taking braces off. That was a great learning opportunity to do what's called the "heavy lifting" of orthodontics and really get confident with it and deal with a variety of challenges. But putting on and taking off braces is not all I learned from Dr. Kott. I also learned practice management from the master.

Dr. Kott's patient base in the northwest suburb of Detroit was a different patient base than I was used to in Ann Arbor. In Dr. Kott's practice, we treated a lot of affluent families in which the parents were extremely involved in their children's treatment. They expected to be informed of and understand every detail of their child's treatment. There was a lot of opportunity for tension between parents and their children and parents and the staff. Observing Dr. Kott, I learned how to be proactive in reading situations and defusing tensions before they became an issue.

A great example occurred when I had arrived just out of residency. Some of the parents had issue with having an orthodontist fresh out of school working on their child, and Dr. Kott preempted their concerns by telling them that I went to the same dental school as he did, and that like him, I was also first in my class, that he had every confidence in me, and that I was going to take good care of their child. Dr. Kott also always took the time to explain the details of the treatment plan, including what problems could arise and how those problems would be addressed if they did occur. The more time I spent in Dr. Kott's practice, the better I understood his reasons for taking the time in the beginning to explain the details in order to eliminate potential areas of contention in the future.

BUYING MY FIRST PRACTICE

As I write this book, I am reminded of the many amazing people with whom I have been fortunate enough to connect along the way. Dr. Keith Wong is one of the great ones. Keith had a significant impact on my journey of self-evolution. But first, let me share the circumstances of our connection.

Keith and I had a very influential person in common, Dr. Lysle Johnston, the chairman of my Orthodontic Department who hired me to teach at Michigan. Dr. Johnston had been the Chairman at the Department of Orthodontics at St. Louis University just a few years prior when Keith had gone there for his specialty degree. It was only three years after I graduated from Michigan that Keith reached out to Dr. Johnston for a recommendation for another partner in his practice, and Dr. Johnston connected him with me. I came up to Lansing from Ann Arbor for an interview with Keith, and it went well. Within two weeks of that interview, Keith's partner in his practice died suddenly. It was tragic and incredibly challenging for all of them. I told Keith that I would come up and help the practice get through, and that at some point, he and I could figure out if my being there was going to work long term or not.

That is how Keith and I first connected, and as I said, he is one of the great ones. Keith has been so influential in my life. I have learned the importance of balance in my life from him. Keith is one of those evolved people who, although they are financially successful, keep their priorities intact, no matter where they are in life. After successfully building a practice, Keith still drove the same beat-up car he was driving in dental school. Material things and status were just not important to him. I remember overhearing a patient's parent say, "Son, don't ever be an orthodontist. Did you see the car Dr. Wong drives? You'll never make any money at it." In a way, Keith was another anchor in my life who taught me how to stay grounded.

Within a year of the loss of his partner, Keith sold the practice to me and moved away. There were three offices involved in the practice, so I sold off two and stayed with the office Keith had been primarily in. This is when the business skills that I had learned from Dr. McNamara and Dr. Kott were invaluable. For the next year, I was the orthodontist, marketer, and practice manager as I navigated my way through owning my own practice.

BUILDING A PRACTICE

One year after purchasing the practice, my now former husband finished his orthodontic residency, and I brought him into the practice as my partner.

The initial two years in the practice (one with Keith and one by myself) were a slow grow for me. Finding the time to get out to meet and greet everyone in the community was a challenge because I was so busy treating patients and managing all the business aspects of the practice. My former husband is naturally social, so when he came on board, he took the lead on building us up in the community. This seemed like a good balance at the time, as we both gravitated toward our strengths. Mine was organization and practice management, and his was business development.

Over the next few years, the partnership worked in terms of establishing a large and successful practice. As a couple and as orthodontists, we were well known in the community, and we had a growing number of patients who would travel a distance to be treated at our practice. All my hard work seemed to be paying off, and between my training, teaching, and practice, I was now a well-respected authority in the field of orthodontics.

Several years into the practice, I noticed that our adult patient population was increasing, especially women. And then more of our female patients began to request to see me. I attribute this to the level of communication that I provide and my ability to empathize with the unique needs of women. In me, they had a practitioner who understood the many responsibilities that we as women take on and have to juggle on a daily basis. By this time, I was not only a professor, businessperson, orthodontist, and wife, but also a mother of two beautiful children.

A WELL-OILED MACHINE

My life was running like a well-oiled machine. Here I was living the life I had worked so hard to achieve, a life that provided me the opportunity to change lives through orthodontics and enjoy a rich family life with my husband and our two children.

Foundation for Treating Adults

Being able to change not just children's lives through orthodontics but also the lives of a growing number of adults was and is a true gift to me. I didn't consciously plan to develop a strong adult patient base. As I have mentioned, the primary focus of orthodontics tends to be children, but when I look back, I realize that I set the foundation for treating adults with my first published paper in 1996. Based on my graduate thesis, my paper addressed the long-term facial-growth changes in people seventeen years old and older. By the age of seventeen, the individual's physical growth is primarily complete. However, through my research, I identified the many changes that continue to occur during adulthood in our facial and bone structures and the soft tissue in our face, lips, nose, and chin.

> **Being able to change not just children's lives through orthodontics but also the lives of a growing number of adults was and is a true gift to me.**

This initial research provided me with a lot of information about how an adult's face changes over the years, which is critical in my treatment of young children. When assessing young children for treatment, I start with the end in mind. I always ask myself, "How will what I do now affect their smile and health in the future?" Because I understand the changes that occur during adulthood, I am in a better position to maximize the long-term aesthetics of a person's smile. It's like bookends: I have the long-term and the early treatment knowledge and experience. This has given me great wisdom in approaching both children and adult patients individually and providing them the best long-term solutions possible.

Juggling It All

The practice was booming, I was married with two beautiful, healthy children, we had a beautiful home, and I continued to teach and accept requests for speaking engagements. Every woman reading this understands how both wonderful and stressful juggling all of life's responsibilities can be, and I was no different. As is my nature, when life was stressful, I found solace in my ability to focus and throw myself into my work. As time went on, I found myself seeking this solace more and more, but it would be a few more years before I realized that my own inner smile had begun to fade.

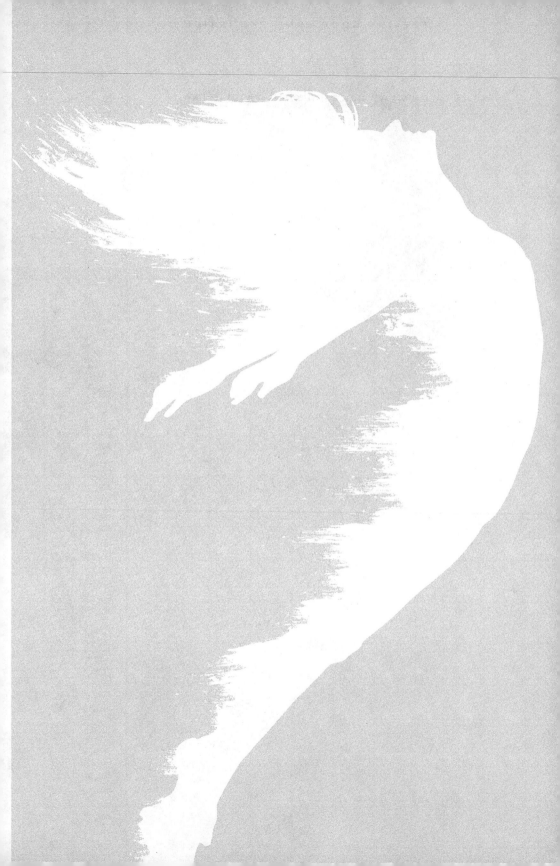

CHAPTER 5

WHEN YOUR INNER SMILE IS UPSIDE DOWN

And the day came when the risk to remain tight in a bud
was more painful than the risk it took to blossom.
—ANAÏS NIN

Looking at my life from the outside, it was everything I had dreamed of. I graduated from orthodontics in 1995, I married in 1997, and I bought my first practice in 1999. In 2000 my husband joined the practice, and we bought a house. We welcomed our first child, Katie, in 2001 and our second child, Will, in 2002. During all that, I was also teaching and practicing part time in Ann Arbor. Such is the life of an overachiever, leaving little time to breathe, let alone time to nurture my own needs.

CRACKS IN THE VENEER

It was near the end of 2009 that I allowed myself to acknowledge the cracks in our beautifully built life. By this time, our practice had grown so big that we were seeing one-hundred-plus patients a day, five days a week, booked out ten to twelve weeks in advance. We had created a monster that we could no longer control. There was no room for flexibility or for more time to spend with our children. We were the only two orthodontists, and we didn't feel like we could turn patients away so we could close for vacation for a week or two throughout the year.

> **When you are in that cycle of focusing on the growth of a business—how many patients can you serve, how much money can you make—it is easy to lose sight of what's real in life.**

It felt to me like the practice owned us. When you are in that cycle of focusing on the growth of a business—how many patients can you serve, how much money can you make—it is easy to lose sight of what's real in life. Life had become a blur.

I cannot pinpoint the defining moment, but somewhere in the blur, I finally found a piece of clarity that jolted me back to reality. As I began to look at my life with objectivity, I realized that I had lost my ability to be compassionate to the real-life challenges that others faced, an ability that I had learned from Dr. McNamara and had purposefully worked to develop over the years. From that point forward, I began the slow and steady process of looking inward, and the clouds gradually began to clear for me. It was only then that I was able to begin my journey back to my path of being a real person who could empathize with what others were going through, and who could nurture my true self.

A CATALYST FOR CHANGE

There is an annual gala, Dancing with the Local Stars, that supports the Carefree Medical and Dental Clinic here in Lansing. In 2009, I was one of the local "celebrities" they asked to participate in the dancing part of the gala. That meant committing to perform a ballroom dance, which also meant committing to training with a professional dancer to learn the dance. It was a considerable time commitment to be sure, and time was something I had so little of. Our new home was in the final stages of being built, we were preparing to move, the kids were busy seven- and eight-year-olds, the practice was flourishing, and I had no time for dancing. I told them I would think about it and let them know.

Over the next few days, my inner voice, that I hadn't listened to in so long, began nagging at me and telling me that I had to do this. And I am not sure why, but after so many years of silencing my inner voice, I decided to listen. I called the clinic back and agreed to dance! The weeks leading up to the gala were busy and exciting, and when I returned home the night of the gala, I was on cloud nine. I was energized and happy in a way that I hadn't been in a very long time, and I realized it was the first time in years I had done something just for me and just for the pure pleasure of it. It was the first time in a long time that my smile inside and outside was almost too big to contain.

Dancing in the gala was the beginning of the end of my life as I knew it. There was still work to be done before I would fully return to my true path—but there was no turning back now.

A NEW PERSPECTIVE

One of the things that training for and dancing in the gala gave me was a space to be me—to simply be Kristine. Not Dr. West, not a wife, not Mom, not a business owner, not a professor, just me. Matt, my dance partner, knew nothing about me. To him I was a woman who wanted to dance; that's it. That simple existence during our dance times is what set me free. That freedom allowed me to step back a bit and view my life from a new perspective.

I began to ask myself, "Where am I, how did I get here, and is this really the life I was looking for?" These questions made me realize that the many compromises I had made over the years for my marriage and for the practice left little room for myself. I had kept my head down working like crazy, making sure my kids, my husband, and our practice were taken care of, and in the midst of it all, I had relinquished room for my own needs. My husband's world had become my world. Little by little I had chosen to give up time with my family and my friends because it was easier to go along than to fight for what I wanted. What had felt balanced in the beginning, me with my nose to the grindstone at the practice and my husband's focus on socializing and community engagement, now felt isolating.

These realizations were terrifying for me because it meant I would have to make a lot of extremely difficult life choices. If my marriage wasn't going to work, what would that mean for my kids, for the practice, for this life I thought I had so carefully built? But the more I peeked beneath the veneer, the more I realized I had arrived at this point for a variety of reasons. At the top of the list was my need to overachieve in order to feel good about myself and to feel OK with my life. It is a need that always leaves you wanting more. I had to learn that once the top grade—the award, the successful practice, whatever it is—is achieved, that's it, it's over, and then you charge onto the next thing and the next, and it is never enough. That level of drive isn't sustainable over time, and I knew I had to learn to let some of that go.

I also had to learn when to quit. I couldn't see how I could get through what I saw as a significant failure—divorce. Quite honestly, part of why I stayed so long was because I wanted to prove to myself that I could have a successful marriage. I wanted to break what I saw as the cycle of my mother's history of difficult relationships. I just didn't want to screw up. I was so committed to proving that I could have a successful marriage that I refused to see how much of myself I was losing in the process.

ON MY OWN

In June 2011, we announced our separation. In the state of Michigan, they require a six-month separation before you can officially file for divorce. That was a strange and difficult time. We were separated but still living in the same house and still working together in the practice.

Over the next several months, I had to extricate myself from my current life and start to create a new one. I chose to leave the practice behind. That was really tough because I had worked so hard to build it, and I loved caring for the patients, and work had always been my solace during times of stress, and now it was no longer there. But I knew I had to make a drastic shift if

> **But I knew I had to make a drastic shift if I was going to come through this better and stronger.**

I was going to come through this better and stronger. I bought a house and began the process of remodeling and making it a home for my kids and me.

One of my challenges during this time was feeling like I was living in a fishbowl. Our private life suddenly seemed so public, and I am a very private person. It felt like everywhere I went when someone would say hi, all I could think was how they knew about the divorce and my leaving the practice. It was difficult for me. I know being on social media is so common today, but for me it is still a struggle to put myself out there in such a public way.

In early 2012, once I sold my share of the practice to my now former husband, and I was out of the marital house and in my own home, I was able to make the time and space for connections that helped me heal. I began riding horses again, I continued with my dancing after the gala, and I reconnected with my biological father, Jerry, and really developed a strong relationship with him during that time. I welcomed the support of my mother and close friends. I had friends and family members say to me, "It's good to have you back. We lost you for a while." And they were right: in the process of losing myself, I had also lost important personal connections.

The best gift through this ordeal was time with my children. I felt like I was making up for lost time, and I welcomed the chance to be fully present when I was with them. That was something I realized I hadn't been very often—present. Life was always a rush of planning, scheduling, and doing with no real time for quiet to just be with each other.

CHAPTER 6

FINDING OURSELVES, FINDING OUR SMILES

*Use your smile to change the world, but don't
let the world change your smile.*
—*UNKNOWN*

My husband and I lived in a community that knew us first and foremost as a couple, and as is with most divorces, there are friends who remain friends and those who feel they need to choose a side. Dr. Steve Powell was a friend to both of us, and thankfully he remained so.

I first met Steve when I'd joined Keith's practice. He had the dental practice next to ours, and he and Keith had built the building both of our businesses were housed in. I got to know Steve early on; sometimes he'd come over in between patients and chat, and then when my husband joined me, Steve befriended him, too, and then we got to know Steve's wife and kids. Steve's friendship was one of the constants that sustained me through the divorce.

Over the years, Steve had told us about a river rafting program that he and his children had participated in. The program's mission was to help parents and their kids connect with each other and help kids (especially teens) find their true path and calling in life. He spoke highly of the program and its leader, Kyle Mercer. Then one day during my separation, Steve and I were out to lunch, and he brought up the program again and said that this same instructor, Kyle, was offering another program that he thought would help me navigate the tumultuous waters I found myself in and help me discover what I needed to do to be true to myself.

TURNING POINT

It was a four-day retreat in upstate New York, and I decided I needed to go. I believe opening myself to that opportunity of dancing in the gala is what enabled me to be open to this new opportunity with Kyle. It was at this point that I had begun to allow myself to veer from the carefully laid tracks that I thought I was supposed to be on. I had no idea what I was getting into, and it was scary. I had always been a planner. Because of my abandonment issues, I always tried to control what I could in my life, to have my plans mapped out so that I knew what was coming next. And now here I was for the first time since I was a young child, at a point in my life where I didn't know what the hell I was going to do. For the first time, I couldn't envision how everything was going to look in the future. It was frightening, but I knew I had to make a change; clearly, what I had been doing was no longer working. I had been running through life so fast that I hadn't given myself a chance to catch up with who I was and what I wanted.

I participated in the retreat with about thirty other people. It was intense. Through journaling, group sessions, and individual sessions, I really worked through and began to let go of a lot of emotional pain. At my last session with Kyle that week, he recognized that I was going through significant changes in my life, and he offered to continue coaching me one-on-one. I said yes. I felt like I was ready to continue the work; I had surrendered myself to the Universe and was open to new pathways. I left the retreat with feelings of freedom and empowerment, and the beginning of acceptance of myself.

The retreat and agreement to continue to counsel with Kyle was my first big step in my journey to evolve and accept myself in this new place in the world. The months of guidance from Kyle helped me look at myself and the world in a whole new way. I learned to let go of the ties and expectations of society, of the people in my life who were not supporting my evolution, and of my own expectations for myself, and to chart a new course untethered by emotions and experiences that had bound and driven me in the past.

CHOOSING ME

The biggest lesson I learned through my self-introspection was to accept that I am not perfect—that my expectation of having to be the best, the number one, the perfect student, orthodontist, wife, mom, daughter, the perfect fill-in-the-blank, was unattainable and unhealthy. I finally reached the point in my evolution when I could take a breath and say, "I don't have to be perfect in order to be loved." I had to learn to love

> We need to fill ourselves with ourselves and nourish our souls and our connections to our higher power rather than expecting others to fulfill us.

myself as I was and accept that in spite of the illusion, we are all alone in the world except for our personal belief in and connection to our Source, God, the Universe. I learned that we need to fill ourselves with ourselves and nourish our souls and our connections to our higher power rather than expecting others to fulfill us. Once we can approach another person with a full version of ourselves (from a place of abundance), rather than as a person who is looking outside to be satisfied or OK (from a place of neediness), then the connection can be one of mutual exchange. To reach this point, I first had to figure out why I had such a need to be perfect, why I had made the choices I did, and how to forgive myself for all of my imperfect choices.

My Achilles' Heel

My drive and my competitive spirit have always been a part of who I am, a part that was fueled and fostered through the instability of my childhood and by my stepdad's "We don't compete to compete; we compete to win and dominate" mentality.

I was always aware of my drive and ambition, and I intentionally cultivated it. I remember in my preteens consciously deciding that because so much in my home life felt out of control, I was going to take charge of my life as much as possible. I was going to live it to the fullest, live it with no regrets, and always be the best I can be. In other words, I was going to take control of as many aspects of my life as I could and be the best at all of them. School was the first arena in which I worked fiercely to be the best. Then there was horseback riding, and even socializing. Yes, I was a competitive socializer! I could never just relax and have a party. I had to blow it out every time; it always had to be a party that was too amazing to forget. And any time I went out with friends, it would be an event!

As I grew, so, too, did my competitive spirit, and it spilled over into all areas of my life. It wasn't until I began processing this with Kyle that I realized my competitiveness wasn't a positive. Up until that point, I believed my drive and need to compete was a strength, that it meant that I was fully engaged in life. Realizing that my drive, my ego had taken control of my life, and that I had created a competitive monster was a life-changing *aha!* moment for me. My drive, it turns out, was my Achilles' heel.

A Better Me

My evolution is a lifelong process. My Achilles' heel didn't suddenly disappear, and still today, it trips me up from time to time. What's different now is that I recognize it for what it is. My drive was my bridge to self-esteem. My self-worth was tied up in victory, in winning, whether it was grades, class ranking, biggest practice, any and all of those things. Striving to be the best, to dominate, was my go-to when I felt left out or insecure, or when a relationship wasn't satisfying my needs. Growing up, schoolwork was my focus for overachieving, and as an adult, when I was feeling unsatisfied or insecure, work—being the best orthodontist, having the biggest practice—was the focus of my drive.

Not engaging in work during the most difficult time of my life, although incredibly painful, was essential to my growth. Work was what I always fell back on to fill me. Now going through this major life change, I really had to rely on myself internally to sustain me rather than always latching onto the external parts that I let define me. Work had been a major anchor in my life, and now I had to release it and learn to anchor myself. Through my work with Kyle, I recognized that my unrelenting drive was unsustainable, and that I had to jump off this racing train I had created. I jumped and felt a bit bruised and broken, but that time of vulnerability gave me space to heal. In that healing, I also became a better parent.

When I met you, you had already made the declaration for your own liberation, freedom, and empowerment, but you hadn't integrated it yet. It seems that the story arc since I have known you has been this growing understanding and integration of your own empowerment and being your own sense of security, being your own sense of rightness, and finding groundedness in yourself rather than outside yourself.
—*KYLE MERCER*

One thing I had after I left the practice was time to myself. Through that quiet time, I became more sensitive to everything that was going on in the world. I can see that the drive I am working so hard to temper is always pushing at us from external forces. Seeing my children go through the college application process, and the fierce push to compete that is so ingrained in that process, is eye-opening. There are parents who push their kids into everything. They spend tens of thousands of dollars on essay-writing coaches. It is so insane, the pressure we put on our kids and ourselves. I think my kids are in a better place because I continue to make the shift away from my own competitiveness. And I have learned so much from them. The truth is my kids are better at not jumping onto the competition train than I am. I have seen them both outright reject the concept.

When it was time for my daughter to choose which college she would attend, initially she was dead set on going to Washington University like me; she was driven to obtain that goal. At some point during the process, she made this shift and decided that attending the big, prestigious school wasn't important to her, that going to a school where she could feel connected and happy was what mattered. She told me that she just wasn't going to play the game. She chose to listen to her inner voice. Because I had made my own shift, I was able to give her the space to follow her intuition and find her own path.

That was an incredible parenting moment for me. I know it hasn't always been easy for them to have such an overachiever for a mother. I'm a much better parent now, but I still have to work on not feeding into the competition game, especially not putting that on them. And seeing my kids choosing to live a grounded and happy life makes my heart as a parent so full.

Learning to Forgive

I have always been really good at beating up myself for making choices in life that I later looked back on and wondered what was I thinking, wishing I had made a different choice. Now when I look back, I take ownership of my choices and accept them for what they are: choices. Sometimes we make good ones, and sometimes we don't. What I do know now is that whatever decision I made in the past, it was the best decision I could make at that moment in my life with the person I was and the knowledge I had. That's it. I can't go back and change it, but I can learn

> I take ownership of my choices and accept them for what they are: choices. Sometimes we make good ones, and sometimes we don't.

from it and become a better, stronger person for it. I forgive myself for my mistakes and my imperfect choices and accept that they were part of what made me who I am today, and I relax around it.

MOVING FORWARD

Once I found my true self, it opened the door for others to see the true me. Scott was one of the first people in my life with whom I thought,

"He really sees me; he sees the true me." Scott and I had met through a mutual friend years ago at a conference. Scott was a regional manager for a prominent orthodontic manufacturing and supply company, and in 2011 our paths crossed again. As we began talking, we shared that we were both going through divorces, and from there we became friends who supported each other through that challenging time.

I think one of the reasons why we hit it off so well was because we didn't really know anything about each other. We were clean slates, and over time, as we leaned on each other during our struggles, we connected on a deep level and eventually began dating. But of course, I never take the easy path. The man I was becoming so deeply involved with lived six hours away. This was another life test that forced me to challenge my natural instincts. I am an action person, always ready to go. But it was important to both of us to make sure life was stable for our respective kids, which meant building our life together gradually. I had to learn to put on the brakes and take a slower path.

My kids and I lived in Michigan, and Scott and his kids lived in New York. We maintained two households even after we married in 2014. It wasn't until August of 2019 that, for the first time, we lived in the same house. I am realizing that every obstacle in life is an opportunity for growth. For someone with abandonment issues, living apart from my significant other was emotionally challenging. There were many times when I didn't think we were going to make it, because I would worry that if I was out of Scott's sight, I was out of his mind. But I also wanted to remain true to focusing on and really being there for my kids during that period. I worked through it. I had a lot of time to myself to facilitate my own development. It was almost like getting myself complete and full before we were together all the time.

CRAFTING A NEW PRACTICE

Eventually in December 2015, through my work with Kyle and a lot of soul searching, it became clear that I needed to open my own solo orthodontic practice and have a place where I could truly deliver the level of orthodontic and interpersonal care that I had always dreamed of. I started crafting my new vision, keeping at the forefront how I wanted patients to feel when they were there.

In starting the practice, I knew there were two critical components. The first was the environment of the practice: I wanted all my patients to be approached from a place of love. My new practice would focus on connecting with each patient, truly hearing them, and meeting them where they were on their journey, right now, that day. My practice would be a sanctuary for my patients to feel at peace. Second, with this practice, I would have full ownership and control of how it moved forward. Starting a practice from scratch would also satisfy another need. Yes, I had learned how to let go of some of my drive, but that didn't mean I had to lose the part of me that loves a challenge, that loves to grow. I still wanted to grow as a professional, a businessperson, and in general as a person.

My drive and my desire to challenge myself are occasionally at odds still. It is like sorting through the clutter and keeping only the good parts. Up to this point, I had accomplished so much in my field. I had practiced in a practice, I had bought into a practice, I had been a partner in a practice, I had owned a practice, I had taught and nationally lectured on orthodontics, and I had done orthodontic research. I felt like the only thing I hadn't done was build a practice from scratch. Why did I want to do it? It's like someone who wants to climb a mountain: because it's there. It was the mountain I hadn't climbed yet. At this point in my life, I felt like I had nothing to lose. I decided I was just going to do it and not look back. My new practice was going to be completely different from my other practices, and it was going to be awesome.

CHAPTER 7

SET YOUR SMILE FREE

Don't forget to dance, no, no, no.

Don't forget to smile.

—*RAY DAVIES*

We all have moments when we are presented with a new opportunity that wakes us up to life, to self-reflection, and to lasting change. For me, that opportunity was ballroom dancing. Although dance has brought me so much joy, I have to admit that my initial introduction to dancing was bittersweet; it was truly what set my inner smile free, but it also made me realize that my life as I knew it was over. Ballroom dancing was the catalyst for my journey of introspection and change.

FIRST STEPS

Our first meeting in preparation for the gala was held at the Carefree Medical and Dental Clinic in Lansing. This was the introductory meeting of the local celebrities and the professional dancers we would be paired with. We were all new to the experience and didn't know each other. When I walked in, I noticed this one dancer, and there was something about him that I was immediately drawn to. You know when you walk into a room, and for some unexplainable reason, you feel an instant connection to a perfect stranger? That's what I felt.

Once we were all seated, the head of the fundraiser began explaining how the entire process worked and what we could expect. Then they announced the pairings. Lo and behold, I was paired with the gentleman whom I had noticed when I first walked in. Matt and I clicked immediately. We introduced ourselves and began to formulate a plan and scheduled time to practice at the studio that Matt danced at. And that's how it all began. I was so excited, and I had no idea what I was doing or what to expect, which is what made the whole experience so beautiful. I went into it completely empty of any expectations or preconceived notions, which I now realize is the best way to approach most things in life: emptying yourself of judgment allows you to freely experience the moment.

The next step was the assignment of the type of dance we would perform. I love all dance, so it didn't really matter to me. But when Matt and I were assigned the Hustle, I was excited, because growing up I was a bit of a closet disco junkie. Disco wasn't very cool with my peer group, so I had to pretend that I only liked bands like KISS and Cheap Trick. It was taboo to talk about the Bee Gees or any disco group. But now, I could celebrate and talk about disco music and dancing because, after all, that's what I had been assigned through no choice of my own! We chose "You Should Be Dancing" by the Bee Gees.

A METAPHOR FOR MARRIAGE

I know so much more about ballroom dancing now, but at the time of the gala, it was all new to me, and because it was a show dance rather than a competitive dance, we weren't tied to a structure. We were able to be free-form, which was perfect because Matt is a modern dancer, which is completely expressive and free-form. Developing our dance routine was a wonderfully creative process; forming a partnership between the two of us with our movements, matching those movements to the music, and creating our overall presentation was freeing and exhilarating.

We began practicing a couple of times a week, and through that process, we developed a lasting friendship. When you dance with someone, it's a metaphor for marriage or for a partnership with anyone. In dance, as in a partnership, you have to be able to move on your own. You have to move yourself, yet you have to maintain a connection with your partner and respond to and move with that person.

You and your partner must work together but still be responsible for your own selves. You cannot just let the other person carry you around, or drag you around, or be the motor for your movements. You are in charge of yourself. You have to move yourself. Even if you do lifts, and you are the one being lifted, you actually lift yourself. You mentally and physically lift your body as your partner is also lifting you.

Matt was such a great partner for me. He was so different from everyone else in my life. He truly is one of a kind, genuinely judgment free, and so much fun to be around. Matt and dance coming into my life at that time were just what I needed. He didn't know me as Dr. West, or as a mom, or a wife. He only knew me as a fellow human being; I was a clean slate, which was another aspect of this experience that helped set me free.

That's how we got started. We performed at the gala and were one of the crowd favorites. We had so much fun. Then, after it was over, it felt like such a letdown of adrenaline, excitement, and joy, so we decided to keep going. We found a dance studio we could practice at, and we began our formal ballroom training.

LEARNING TO SMILE AGAIN

Ballroom dancing was new to both of us. That made it a little more challenging, because the ideal scenario for an amateur couple would be for one to dance with a female pro and learn the male part, and the other person to dance with a male pro and learn the female part, and then the amateur couple would come together and know how to sync up. We were a bit like the blind leading the blind, which honestly, I think made it more fun, forced me to take it slower, and enabled me to enjoy the journey rather than focus on an end goal.

Over the next two years, Matt and I trained with Louis, the head dance pro at the studio, and his stepson, Gage. Louis was a top ballroom competitor in the country, and Gage had just turned pro a few years prior to that time. During this period, Matt and I did a couple of showcase dance recitals at the studio, but primarily we focused on training in preparation for competitive ballroom dancing.

Those two years dancing with Matt made me realize how much my inner smile had diminished. I can still remember that feeling of joy when it was time to go to the studio and dance, to feel that part of me reignited. It created a fire in me that I hadn't felt in an awfully long time.

I still loved my work. I was always a hard worker, and that didn't suddenly stop. Heck, I was voted hardest worker in my high school senior class. No one outworks me. I no longer think of that as the badge of honor that I thought it was in high school, and a lot of that shift in thought is due to my experience with dance. Dancing allowed me to step out of my existence a few hours a week. I began to realize that I had created a life that was so structured, so planned out, that it felt like I was playing this role in a life that I was no longer scripting. Dance provided me an escape from that role, and with that came objectivity.

Over time, I had given bits of myself away while I was busy taking care of everyone else. Dance was finally something I was doing just for me, and it started to really change my outlook on my life and how I viewed myself. Through dance, I began to grow as an individual again. Through that evolution, I reached a point when I realized that there was no room in my current life for me to be fully in my own existence. There started to be this dichotomy, where the person that I truly am, and that I wanted to continue to be, was like a phoenix rising from the ashes. That person couldn't reconcile how to remain in my current life situation; I could not make it mesh any longer.

> **I began to realize that I had created a life that was so structured, so planned out, that it felt like I was playing this role in a life that I was no longer scripting.**

One day I just imploded. It was early 2011, and I was out of town with my girlfriend Jean. We were out to dinner, and I just literally had a breakdown. I began sobbing and asking, "Who am I? How did

I get here?" and saying, "This is not the life that I wanted." I knew I couldn't force it to work anymore and that I had painful decisions to make. I think that my experience in dance and with Matt connected me so deeply with myself that I was able to gain the strength to make the changes in my life that needed to be made.

As I was making major changes in my life, so, too, was Matt. In the late summer of 2011, he announced that he was moving to California. I was deeply saddened by the news. Matt leaving felt like another significant loss, because he had become such an important part of my life. But at the same time, it was important for me to support him in his life's journey to go out into the world and experience new places and people.

So there I was, newly separated, preparing to move into a new house, saying goodbye to Matt, and soon-to-be no longer working. This was a time of major changes, and I had to find a new way of adapting, because I would no longer have my work to bury myself in. I knew I had to keep dancing. That summer, Gage and I started dancing as a Pro-Am (professional-amateur) couple, and things just took off from there. In April 2012, I was ready for my first big competition.

GETTING UNCOMFORTABLE

Preparing for my first competition, I was so nervous. In fact, I had terrible stage fright for the first four or five years—that's right, *years*. Every time I took that first step onto the dance floor, I would literally shake. Stage fright felt ridiculous to me. I've lectured at national meetings, I've been lecturing to orthodontic students for over twenty years, I talk in front of groups frequently, but for some reason, I had such stage fright when dancing. The nerves took me by surprise. But in retrospect, I think it was all the unknowns. I wasn't used to unknowns. After all, I'm the person who planned every detail of her life. The first competition was especially nerve-racking; I had absolutely no idea what to expect, and I had to just had to drop the reins and let things happen.

When you prepare for competition, there is more to do than practice dancing. When you first start, you have to rely on your pro to guide you in getting your hair and makeup done, your costumes and jewelry picked out and ready, and even your spray tan. Once I learned the ropes, I was able to manage all the preparations, but not the stage fright. For the first couple of dances, I would always feel myself shaking, but then I would relax and be able to go with the flow.

I didn't let the unknowns and the nerves stop me. I was at a point in my life where I was actively seeking to enrich myself, and to do that you have to put yourself in uncomfortable situations in order to grow. I was no longer going to be just a mom, a wife, an orthodontist … and then that's it: no identity that was just mine. And I know I am not alone in this revelation. I think there are a lot of women my age who are searching for the same thing, whether they are fully aware of it or not.

One of my college roommates learned to play the harp when she was in her forties. Mary wanted to enrich her life, so she took up the harp, and now she plays with an ensemble in Philadelphia, which I think is amazing. She said that for a long time, she used to throw up every time right before she went on stage. That made me realize that my stage fright was normal and, more importantly, that it was OK to feel nervous. The more I learned to own my stage fright, to acknowledge and accept it, the more comfortable I became, and the stage fright gradually diminished over time.

REFRAMING MY COMPETITIVE SPIRIT

Now the time to compete had arrived, and competing is something I have always excelled at. In ballroom dance competitions, everyone enters at the bronze level, and the highest level is open, with silver and gold being in between. And within each level are distinct categories like pre-bronze, intermediate, advanced, and full bronze. And within those categories, dancers are grouped by a ten-year age bracket such as forty-five to fifty-four.

Dance competitions are usually three to four days in length, with each style being done on one day; this way dancers can have their hair, makeup, and costumes created to complement that style of dance. American rhythm and smooth are on different days, as are international ballroom and Latin. Finally, the time arrives for your turn, and you and your partner step onto the dance floor, and they cue you as to the type of dance. For example, they would say, "OK, cha-cha music, please." The music plays, and you do your cha-cha. Then you have about fifteen seconds, and then they announce the next dance that you will do. Everyone in your group is moving across the floor, navigating around each other while trying to dance to the rhythm of the music.

On rhythm day, for example, dancers do five unique style dances in a row, and then the round is over. Sometimes you step off the floor until your next round of dances comes up, or perhaps you stay on the floor to continue to compete. I have been at competitions at which I have done thirty heats/dances in a row without stepping off the floor for a break! The process is orchestrated down to the smallest detail. It can be two to three days of nonstop dancing. There have been some weekends that Gage and I have danced upward of 150 heats.

It's no secret that I love to win. I always have, and I always will, but what I learned from ballroom dancing is that doing something for the win and doing something for the pure joy of it are two vastly different things. The high you get from winning is fleeting, but when you experience pure joy, that's a feeling that stays with you.

I remember one of my mentors, Dr. Lysle Johnston, who was the chairman of the Orthodontic Department at Michigan while I was a resident and is still a world-renowned orthodontic instructor and researcher, told me, "You don't need awards and recognition to validate what you've done. If you lose, don't read too much into it. If you win, don't read too much into it." His wisdom really resonated with me at this juncture in my life. It helped me to remain neutral about the competitive aspect of dancing and allowed me to dance for the pure joy of it.

Lysle's words of wisdom were not the only ones that ushered me along this path. As in my world of orthodontics, I also met amazing people in my new world of ballroom dance who offered me guidance. Art and Betty are two of those people. They had been dancing as an amateur couple for over thirty years, and they took lessons in the same studio that Gage and I did. Art and Betty are both retired psychologists. Art is in his late eighties and still competing! They were both always offering me encouragement, and I shared with them my struggles with the competition and about my stage fright.

Art said, "Listen, dance is different. Like me, you are used to studying hard, working hard, and getting the results. Dance is not like that. Often with dance, the harder you work at it, the fewer positive results you will see. You almost have to work less." Then he shared with me that he used to have terrible stage fright, and like me, he felt it was ridiculous because he was successful in all aspects of his life and was comfortable speaking to groups. But one day on the dance floor, he realized that winning or not winning the dance competition didn't have any significant impact on his life. He told me, "At that point I thought, 'Who the hell cares,' and I went out and danced better than I'd ever danced before."

I try to no longer let the high of win or the low of loss corrupt my frame of my mind or my enthusiasm. I have found that the more I let go and don't focus so hard on winning, the more joy comes to me. It is something I am always working on as a recovering overachiever. I now try to notice when these emotions or my drive comes up, and then I acknowledge them and relax around them. Every dance competition becomes an arena for me evolve and radiate my inner and outer smiles.

When one competes and performs on the dance floor, one of the best things you can do is to smile while you dance. Contrary to how it sounds, this is not easy to do. To hold a smile on your face without straining is physically challenging. In fact, I remember one of my high school friends, Bonnie, who was always very peppy and cheerful, decided to enter a smiling contest at our local shopping mall. I was there with a few of our friends to support her. The regulations were that you had to have at least a few of your teeth showing, and your lips could never come together. With her facial muscles twitching at the end, she pulled off the win!

Performing on the dance floor with a smile on your face and truly enjoying yourself is a very important advantage when you are being judged. There have been times when I have scored higher than a dancer who was equally or more skilled than I just because I was smiling and more enjoyable to watch. I now love coming off the dance floor and having people come up to me and say, "I love watching you dance! You are so much fun to watch, and you look like you are having a great time!" To me this is what I will take away as my biggest success in dancing, because the smile that I have found inside me again I can share with the world and really make an impact on others. Everyone has this ability inside them, and once you unleash this powerful way to connect with others, it can be life-changing for you and for those around you—even people you do not know.

Gage and I remained at the bronze level for four years. It is not uncommon for dancers to stay in a category for a few years, but for me, who always believed that "we don't compete to compete; we compete to win," to be able to genuinely enjoy the process even though I wasn't constantly racking up the wins and or moving up the levels with lightning speed was tremendous personal

> **Everyone has this ability inside them, and once you unleash this powerful way to connect with others, it can be life-changing for you and for those around you—even people you do not know.**

growth. I have been dancing at the silver level since 2016 and love the challenges it brings through more advanced choreography and movement. Through competitive ballroom dancing, I learned to reframe my competitive spirit.

CHAPTER 8

GET THE SMILE YOU WANT

It was only a sunny smile, and little it cost in the giving, but like the morning light it scattered the night and made the day worth living.
—*F. SCOTT FITZGERALD*

Finding empowerment through something like I did with dance is great, but when it comes to finding your smile, modern dentistry is truly a world of miracles. Whatever you don't like about your teeth can be changed. If you want them bigger, whiter, straighter, you got it. Always keep in mind that the perfect smile is not perfect. Over-the-top perfection isn't the aim. The aim is always a natural smile.

A NATURAL SMILE

There are studies that have been done for many years on what makes a smile attractive. Even in the past twenty-five years since I was a resident, there has been a shift in what is categorized as a "textbook" beautiful smile. If you look at a group of people who have never had braces, and whose teeth fall into place as they naturally should, you will find common denominators. Among these commonalities are teeth that are straight and not rotated, lining up in a natural arc or curve, the front top teeth overlapping the front lower teeth a couple of millimeters, and the gingival contours of the front teeth being symmetric right to left in what we in the profession know as high-low-high. We know certain things about what is natural. To me, teeth are "German engineered." I say that because every cusp and every fossa or every dip in the tooth is there for a reason. Each tooth has a different anatomy, and the anatomy is specific, so teeth need to align properly with their counterparts on the opposite arch. How your teeth fit together is like the pieces of a jigsaw puzzle.

Many adults who come in are unhappy with their smiles. They don't always know what isn't right, but they know something is off. It could be that their teeth are different lengths or their gumlines are uneven due to the wearing down of their teeth. It is my goal to make their smiles as youthful and natural as possible, which might mean providing a little tooth movement to lift the teeth or establishing that high-low-high gingival relationship for the front upper teeth, thereby allowing the dentist to restore the original length of their teeth. These adjustments make a major difference in the aesthetics of a smile.

For adults who have never had their teeth sitting together properly but haven't been negatively impacted by it in any significant way, you don't necessarily want to disrupt the system and force the teeth into a new relationship without good reason. With adults, orthodontists must be careful not to overtreat them and create more problems than they had when they came in. Sometimes people will say, "I don't want a braces smile." A "braces smile" means that an orthodontist has overpowered the system and forced teeth to move into unnatural and sometimes unattractive angles.

It's important for orthodontists to work with clear aligners or braces and wires to find the proper balance for that person, to treat within the realm of that person's individual musculature and physiology. It's like the best plastic surgery is one that you can't tell it was done. That's kind of what we want to do with orthodontic treatment. As an orthodontist, I want my patients' teeth and smiles to look so natural and appealing that no one can tell they had treatment and that people just notice their beautiful smiles.

The natural smile is easier to accomplish with children because we are able to work with them while their jaws are still growing. In this way, we can make adaptations in tandem with the natural growth process, rather than changing an existing pattern.

EARLY ORTHODONTIC SCREENINGS AND CARE

As I mentioned in chapter 3, the American Association of Orthodontists recommends that children be screened by an orthodontist at age seven. It's important to have children come in at a young age for a screening so we can assess how their jaws are growing and how their teeth are coming in. We want to catch any issues as early as possible so we can work with them while they're still growing. We don't want to wait until they're older and have developed a full growth-pattern issue. Seven years old is the optimal time in a person's growth and development to create more space in their mouths and make structural adjustments to prevent having to extract any permanent teeth later and prevent avoidable dental work as an adult.

The most common underlying growth problem with children is a lack of growth in the transverse dimension of the upper jaw, what is called a maxillary constriction. The jaws grow in three dimensions—up and down, front to back, and side to side. The transverse dimension is the side to side. We measure this dimension across the roof of your mouth. When you have a constricted (or narrow) upper jaw, which can be a result of genetics, function, or even chronic mouth-breathing, it can cause a whole host of issues.

One of the issues that can occur is what we call a posterior crossbite. This occurs when the top teeth bite inside of the bottom teeth, which is the reverse of how they should be. It can cause significant crowding in the upper jaw, so teeth aren't able to erupt naturally, and they can become impacted. Another significant issue that occurs is a restricted airway, which can cause its own host of problems, including sleep apnea. If these issues are not addressed early, and a jaw is left constricted into adulthood, they can lead to long-term health problems, and eventually the narrow jaw can only be corrected by surgery.

> **Orthodontics can't change genetics, but there are things we can do to help guide an area of growth.**

Another concern we want to catch early is an underbite. This is a growth pattern where the lower jaw is growing in front of the upper jaw. If growth guidance can be started early, there's an excellent chance that the patient can avoid jaw surgery later. There are some things that are genetic, or a family trait, like Jay Leno's strong chin. Orthodontics can't change genetics, but there are things we can do to help guide an area of growth. It comes down to really looking where the child is in the normal range of skeletal development for their age.

Even though the recommended age is seven, I don't always first see patients at seven. I might not see a child for the first time until they are thirteen. For those kids who have a significant issue and we've missed that window of opportunity, it can make it harder to correct because they're that much further down the road in their growth. It's like life; the further you veer off your path, the harder it is to get back on.

Most children will not need early treatment, so our job is to screen and then get out of the way and monitor as needed. If a child is referred to me and they don't need anything, I don't treat them. As a parent myself, I want to make sure the parents who come to me with their kids know that I will treat their kids like I would my own. I will never do something that I wouldn't do for my own children. I stress this practice with my students, telling them, "If a patient walks in your door and does not need treatment, tell them that."

TREATMENT OPTIONS FOR CHILDREN

Rapid Maxillary Expanders

Rapid maxillary expanders are commonly used with children who have a skeletal constriction of the upper jaw. A Rapid Maxillary Expander (RME) is an appliance that is fixed to the child's upper teeth and expands the jaw with the use of a screw that is turned daily with a simple key. Typically, these expanders are a "one-size-fits-all," but I've modified and created my own design so that there is a smaller one for kids under ten, and another one for kids between the ages of eleven and sixteen.

> **Early intervention is like building a house: you need to establish a solid foundation to build upon.**

Early intervention is like building a house: you need to establish a solid foundation to build upon. And if there's a true skeletal problem that goes untreated, you're building a house of cards on a weak foundation. If teeth are not aligning as they should, something as simple as chewing will strain the system, and at some point, the strain will be too great, possibly resulting in jaw joint issues, the fracture of teeth, or even gum and bone loss.

Invisalign First and Invisalign Teen

Invisalign First is a clear aligner system for kids who still have baby teeth. I have used these on kids who are unable to use the expanders for one reason or another. Once kids have reached adolescence and all their permanent teeth are in, then we look at Invisalign Teen as an alternative to traditional braces.

Traditional Braces

Metal braces, wires, and elastics are still used in orthodontic treatment. The classic metal braces are brackets that are attached to the teeth, and then the wire connects the brackets and moves the teeth. Although the technique has not changed much over the years, the brackets themselves are a bit smaller now, and they have aesthetic tooth-colored braces that blend into your natural tooth color.

The other improvement is that the wires are more high-tech. When I began practicing, there were still treatment techniques where the wires that we used had to be bent at the spots of each tooth with precision with the patient in the chair. It was a time-consuming process. Although there is often a need to do detailing bends in the final wires to finish a patient's treatment and smile, the memory wires frequently used today are high-tech. They are made in the shape of a curve, like an arc or an arch, and retain their shape while moving the teeth—these wires can provide a gentler force when used correctly. Back when I had braces, they used what was called heavy intermittent force. Today we use low continuous force, which is much more comfortable for the patient. Now, when braces are first put on, they may be a little uncomfortable for a day or two but not at the level of discomfort that occurred with the heavy force technique of my adolescence, and the adjustments are usually painless.

TREATMENT OPTIONS FOR ADULTS

Aligners, or a type of thinner clear retainers, are the most used orthodontic treatment for adults. Invisalign is the brand-name aligner that most people are familiar with.

With Invisalign, I can treat the case virtually on the computer. I move the teeth on a virtual 3-D platform and then see where to start, where to finish, and what the full treatment process will look like and then make any adjustments needed before I even start the actual treatment. It is a morphing program. You establish how to get the teeth from point A to point Z and then divide it into little steps, and every step is a new set of aligners. With every change of aligner, you're doing a little tooth movement to get the teeth to the final point. The Invisalign process takes on average twelve to eighteen months. During that period, depending on the circumstances and how well the patient is following the plan, I will need to see patients about every three to four months. If there are restorative needs after treatment is complete, that can be done with their dentist.

I explain to all my patients using Invisalign when they view their virtual treatment plan on the computer: "This is a simulation. It's a cartoon of reality. It doesn't necessarily mean everything's going to be *exactly* like that when we're done, so that's why I have to watch you."

Even with this 3-D virtual technology, I still have to be hands-on and closely monitor a patient's progress. I am a highly experienced orthodontist, but I can still be fooled into thinking teeth will progress one way and have them progress another. I have treated big, muscular men whose teeth move as smoothly as a hot knife through butter. And then I've treated petite females whose teeth just won't budge, and it's like moving a mountain. I have learned to not assume anything.

Beware of do-it-yourself aligner treatments through mail-order companies. As I mentioned previously, orthodontic treatment needs to be closely monitored by a trained orthodontist. I have had many patients come to me to fix the damage that a do-it-yourself aligner program has done. Initially, it may seem cost effective, but in the end the patient often needs additional work with an orthodontist to undo the damage.

VIRTUAL TREATMENT

The writing of this book has taken place in the midst of the COVID-19 pandemic, which has thrust a myriad of changes upon how we all function. At my practice, we quickly jumped into virtual consultations as a result. During the time of closure, I began doing virtual consultations with new patients and virtual checkups with existing patients. These types of virtual connections are here to stay, and I think it's great because people are already too busy. For instances where I only need to visually look at how things are fitting, like the aligners, and I don't have to do anything hands-on for that patient, we will accommodate our patients virtually, whether that is a video meeting or through the review of photos the patient sends us through our secure platform. If there is any problem, or the patient prefers to come into the office, we will of course see them in person.

Finding and loving your smile often involves more than having just pretty teeth. If a person is ashamed of their teeth, they may actively refrain from smiling or hold their hand in front of their mouth when they smile. Often, doing something tangible, like orthodontics, to bring out someone's ability to smile confidently, can be a first step toward expressing or sharing their smile. Once the resistance to smile is removed, then the joy of sharing and connecting with others through one's smile is unleashed, and the path to rediscover their inner smile is wide open.

CONCLUSION

DON'T FORGET TO DANCE

Everyone smiles in the same language.
—GEORGE CARLIN

As I write this conclusion, I find myself in a period of overwork and high stress. What's different now when I arrive at these times in my life than, say, ten or even five years ago is that I can reach into my toolbox of techniques, resources, and wisdom that I have collected throughout my journey to help me regroup and refocus. My first step is going to be to step out of it and acknowledge the whirlwind without resisting it. Sometimes that is all that is needed to let the dust settle and be able to observe with clarity what is happening. I have learned from experience that if you are in a whirlwind with everything swirling around you and you find yourself just grabbing at everything flying by, it creates more chaos—you need to step out of that energy in order to gain perspective.

Stepping out of it for me right now means taking a couple of days off work. Taking time from the office can still be a challenge for me. It is still easy for me to fall back into my old workaholic mode if I am not careful, but I remind myself that none of my current stresses involve urgent life-or-death issues. My next step is to remind myself of practices that help me maintain balance and calm over the long haul and then practice them regularly. For me that includes getting physical exercise (ballroom dance being my number-one go-to), doing mindfulness and deep breathing exercises, spending relaxed or fun time with my husband and/or my kids, taking Epsom salt baths, and reading a good book. I know that a combination of these steps will rejuvenate me and enable me to return to work with a calmer, more open mindset.

> **I want to be honest about the fact that staying the course, walking my true path, is not a one-and-done proposition; it is a lifelong process.**

I share these details with you because I want to be honest about the fact that staying the course, walking my true path, is not a one-and-done proposition; it is a lifelong process. It takes work and a toolbox you can reach into for help along the way. I encourage you to develop your own personal toolbox to help keep your inner smile bright. For everyone that toolbox will be different, but I'll offer a few suggestions to get you started:

- Don't be afraid to go against social conventions.

- Listen to and trust your inner voice—then take action!

- Forgive yourself. Accept that whatever decision you made in the past, it was the best decision you could make at that moment in your life with the person you were and the knowledge you had.

- Get physical! Physical activity increases the level of endorphins, which are mood-enhancing hormones.

- Find something that you want to do for the pure joy of it—then do it often.

- Consider working with a life coach or counselor to get help if you feel overwhelmed.

- Look to prayer, meditation, or connection to God or Source to help you find your strength to move past the discomfort required to achieve your higher levels.

- Recognize when it is time to drop the reins and relinquish control.

- Be your own anchor.

- Smile often; it has so many benefits. According to *Psychology Today*, a smile can do the following:[4]

  - Elevate your mood and create a sense of well-being

  - Induce more pleasure in the brain than chocolate

  - Lead to a mood boost even if your smile is forced. As Buddhist author Thich Nhat Hanh said, "Sometimes your joy is the source of your smile, but sometimes your smile can be the source of your joy."

  - Make you seem courteous, likable, and competent

  - Be contagious

---

4   "The 9 Superpowers of Your Smile," Psychology Today, Meg Selig, Changepower, posted May 25, 2016, https://www.psychologytoday.com/us/blog/changepower/201605/the-9-superpowers-your-smile

The most significant lesson I have learned in my search for my inner smile, and one I hope you, as the reader, will take away from my story, is that no one else is in charge of your well-being—that's all you. And just as important, except for parenting, you are not responsible for the well-being of others. If you look outside yourself for happiness, for security, for peace, those needs will never be satisfied. It always comes back to your inner smile.

No one else is in charge of your well-being—that's all you.

Only you can find and nurture your inner smile. When you do that, you become your own anchor, your own source of fulfillment, which puts you in a place of acceptance—acceptance that there will always be things in your life that are out of your control, and acceptance of your whole self, even the parts that you might not like.

This level of self-fulfillment is a hard place to get to. And even when we get there, we don't necessarily stay there. It is always a work in progress. It is made more difficult because as a society, we're all trained to look outside ourselves for happiness, whether it's a new car, a bigger house, or a closet full of shoes. We are a society of *more*, and sometimes it can feel like you are swimming upstream. But for me, I can tell you it has been worth the work.

I know that ten years ago, if I were faced with the same stresses that I am faced with in this moment, I would not have been able to step away and press pause to refresh. Without the years of work I have done with myself, I would have pushed myself to the edge. I would have reverted back to working twelve-hour days, six days a week. It is only now in retrospect that I realize I would have pushed myself to the edge in order to maintain the illusion of control—the illusion that if I work hard enough, if I keep striving for perfection, I will be able to control everything in my life. Now that I no longer buy into the illusion, I live a freer life, and you can too.

ACKNOWLEDGMENTS

I'm only a vessel for all I've learned and unlearned. I take no credit.
—KYLE MERCER

This book is a result of my reflection of my evolution and my journey up until now, and the result of all of the interactions that I have had with others along the way. As I move through life, I see more clearly how key friends and mentors have entered at just the "right" time to support me or guide me through the ups and the downs. I truly believe that this is not unique to me, that every single individual has and will continue to have those kinds of important relationships.

I approach life from the mindset of the perpetual student. I have always found solace through this approach, and I have learned something about myself and my life from all of those whose life journeys have synchronized with mine at one point or another. Various challenges I have met in my past were made surmountable and at times even enjoyable with the help of my friends and my mentors. I acknowledge the many key people who have been supportive of me along the way.

From my childhood years to present time, I recognize those

friends with whom I have spent valuable parts of my life (in a somewhat chronological order): Dr. Linda Mueller, Cretia DiBartolo, Drs. David and Laurie Lockman, Dr. Maria VonderHaar, Mary Kelso Bryson, Mark Dehnert, Howard Demsky, Mark Schactman, Dr. David Plurad, Nancy Koff, Caroline Hu, Karyn Polak, Dr. Jim Webb, Dr. Jeff Walker, Anne Walker, Dr. Calvin Wilson, Dr. Tom Weyrich, Dr. Marcia Harrer Sobek, Dr. Mary Knappenburger, Dr. Jim McNamara, Dr. Lysle Johnston, Dr. Pat Nolan, Dr. David Kott, Dr. Jean McGill, Dr. Burt Hagler, Dr. Tim Hannigan, Dr. Andy Cedarbaum, Dr. Mart McLellen, Dr. Gary Carter, Dr. Steve Scott, Dr. Eric Hannapel, George and Sue Allen, Ellen Sorenson-Lacombe, Dr. Keith Wong, Dr. Steve Powell, Dr. Christine Tenaglia, Dr. Charlotte Cortis, Dr. Laurie Hult, Dr. Sue Popovich, Matt Bebermeyer, Gage Clark, Kim Nurenburg, Susan Dec, Richard Sneary, Rebecca Klinger, Bridget and Ric Balesky, Laura and Chris Nugent, Dr. Alexis Tessler, and Kathi Mitchell. You have all made an indelible mark on my life and I treasure the friendships and the memories.

I want to extend a special thank you to Kierstin Miner-Sabec, who was my children's nanny, and who started working with me when my daughter Katie was only six weeks old. Kierstin was a real-world Mary Poppins and was literally the extension of me in my parenting life, in that she did a major amount of the weekday care giving to my children. She did so many things with them as they grew up that I just was unable to do because of my extreme work schedule. She baked, did crafts, dressed them up for Halloween parties and outings, did hair and makeup for Katie's dance recitals, took them to a myriad of sports activities and lessons, went on field trips with them, spent time in their classrooms, took them to different child-friendly places in mid-Michigan, and basically helped raise them. She is still a significant person in our family and even with a family of her own to focus on, she keeps a close relationship with Katie and my son Will.

With appreciation and deep respect, I also want to thank Kyle Mercer for all of his love, support, and the hours and hours of work he did with me through the Inquiry Method. Through my work with him I have awakened to what it means to be fully present in life. I have learned that my ego and my thoughts are not who I am; my true path is one to be honored and nurtured daily; and most importantly, I have learned the value of letting go of the illusion of control—I finally am able to drop the reins, take full responsibility for my wellbeing and happiness, and live.

A tip of the hat as well to all of the team members I've worked with both at my current practice and those I've worked with at previous practices. Because of your support I was and am able to do my best work for my patients.

I also would like to honor my family, who have been inspirations to me in a variety of ways. It is my mom, Dr. Joyce West, who was my main female role model—from her I learned how to be an accomplished woman in what was for years a male-dominated world. She taught me how to persevere in the face of challenge—even when faced with what could seem an insurmountable challenge—with humility and grace, and sometimes humor.

From my dad, Jerry Imming, I have learned the power of a positive attitude and the power of connecting with others and with family. He passed suddenly on January 8, 2021, but he lived every single day as wholeheartedly as he could. It is astounding how many lives he positively touched. He showed up fully in every interaction he had, be it with friends, family, or even with people he had just met. I'm still learning things from him even now, and I imagine I will be for years to come.

My stepmom, Barb Imming, is one of the kindest people I have ever met: she has the gift of being able to make everyone around her feel welcome and cared for, no matter what the setting is, and this is what I would call "life hospitality."

I would like to acknowledge my stepdad, Dr. W. Dean West, who brought me into the world of dental medicine and who taught me the importance of excellence in your daily work and the art of positive patient interaction.

I appreciate the love and support of the entire Imming family and of my brothers, Christopher and Patrick Imming, and their respective wives Abby and Jen, along with my niece, Claire, and nephews, Henry and Sam. They have given me the extended family I have always dreamed of.

I also want to remember my late Uncle Jim, and my Grandpa and Grandma Spring, whose loving support was my foundation during my earliest years. I also want to acknowledge my Aunt Paula Spring, an accomplished journalist, and my cousin Megan, who were both a part of my younger years.

I want to mention the whole new family that I gained when I married Scott, especially my stepchildren Jack and Katherine, and my niece and nephew, Reilly and Quinn.

I want to lovingly honor my daughter and son, Katie and Will. I am blessed to have been given the gift of being their mom—I have learned so much about myself through my connection with them and through seeing myself through their eyes. When they were born, I was shown the higher purpose of being a parent—suddenly one's focus turns away from oneself toward the wellbeing of one's children. Through trial and error, I parented them and as much as I taught them, I also learned from them.

From Katie I learned the value of noncompetiveness—she showed me how one can excel yet be collaborative with peers. Unabashed and fully owning who she is and what her life is, Katie is grounded in her truth and I truly admire that.

From Will I have learned the value of good sportsmanship and compassion for others. A friend to everyone, he can connect with others of all ages (from two to ninety-five!) and instantaneously make one feel special and at ease, and I commend him for bringing that ability into all aspects of his life. Furthermore, I honor them both for having such strength and clarity of self as they move from their teenage years into their adult years.

And finally I appreciate my husband, Scott Annable, for all of the unwavering love, support, and encouragement he has shown me on my journey to fully becoming Kris. I love being married to him. It is with him that I have been most free to be me.

With love and gratitude,
Kris

ABOUT THE AUTHOR

Dr. Kristine West is a mom, partner, friend, ballroom dancer, and orthodontist who has helped her patients achieve their best outer smiles for over thirty years. At a pivotal moment in her life, Dr. West realized that, although her outer smile shone bright, her inner smile had lost its spark. It was then that she began her journey of introspection and stillness that taught her to once again trust her intuition, listen to her inner voice, and reignite her inner smile. Dr. West lives in Michigan.

CPSIA information can be obtained
at www.ICGtesting.com
Printed in the USA
JSHW031231130421
13534JS00008B/217

9 781642 251814